DATE DUE

Move It!

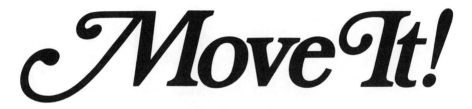

Move It!

Proven Exercises
for Family Health
and Fitness

Phyllis C. Jacobson
Barbara Vance

Bookcraft
Salt Lake City, Utah

Library of Congress Catalog Card Number: 78-67219
ISBN O-88494-357-7

First Printing, 1978

Lithographed in the United States of America
PUBLISHERS PRESS
Salt Lake City, Utah

Contents

Preface

The Livewells reside in a modest three-bedroom house in a suburban community seven miles from the city where Michael Livewell, thirty-seven, has worked as a bus driver for the transit authority for the past seventeen years. Michael and his wife, Sharon, thirty-four, were married soon after they graduated from high school. Sharon is a homemaker who is kept busy as the PTA president in the local elementary school where Timmy, nine, attends fourth grade, and his sister, Michelle, five, attends kindergarten each afternoon. Sharon also works as a volunteer at the community hospital one afternoon a week when all the children are in school. An older daughter, Tina, thirteen, is an eighth grader in junior high school. Jon, sixteen, is in the tenth grade in high school. He recently received a Presidential Sports Award for playing basketball a total of fifty hours, at least fifteen of which had to be in organized junior varsity games (he is a member of the junior varsity basketball squad at school), and of which no more than one hour of basketball per day counted in the total of fifty hours.

Michael drives to work each day in an ancient foreign import car he has owned for twelve years. He usually watches television after dinner, unless it is his weekly league bowling or bridge night, when he and Sharon and three other couples meet on a rotating basis at each other's homes. Sharon, an excellent cook, often complains to her friends that she is putting on weight but hates to diet. Michael is definitely getting a middle-aged spread.

The Livewells represent some of the typical problems American families face in developing a life-style that will help them achieve and maintain fitness. Michael has a job that requires sitting most of the day.

Even when he gets home, he does not engage in activities that require vigorous bodily exertion. His wife, Sharon, is the typical homemaker who is busy all day and fatigued at the end of the day from daily routine but never engages in activity vigorous enough to increase her physical fitness level. The children are active but not involved in a consistent program of physical activity that will help them achieve and maintain a high level of fitness.

What is physical fitness? In general, it is a state of physical well-being. What does this mean? It means your body allows you to engage in all life's activities without undue strain, pain, or fatigue to your muscles and joints. This means every cell of your body is functioning at its highest potential. You have more energy and enthusiasm for work and play. Your body is fortified against disease and less likely to sustain physical injury. Even social relationships are improved and enhanced when bodies are in top shape.

Physical fitness is not only a priceless asset now, but a heritage to be passed from generation to generation. Physically fit parents tend to produce healthy children. Families who maintain a life-style that includes vigorous activity on a continuing basis not only develop physically fit bodies, but also tend to develop close, open relationships with one another and develop family bonds and traditions that are passed on through generations.

This book is written to help families develop these priceless assets. Achieving physical fitness need not be drudgery nor painful. The chapters in this book provide simple, individualized procedures that all family members can follow, but which do not require long periods of preparation nor great expense. The suggested activities can be done in or near any home by the family as a group. Engaging in activities for fitness can be a satisfying, fun experience for all family members, as each person pushes his or her body toward ever-increasing levels of physical achievement.

This book emphasizes flexibility, strengthening, and cardiovascular endurance activities. A minimum level of flexibility and strength is necessary to effectively engage in vigorous activity to develop cardiovascular endurance. Therefore, Part One helps you assess how flexible and strong your body is now and how to plan a program that will get you from where you are to where you want to be. Part Two is designed to teach you how to assess your level of cardiovascular endurance and how to plan and implement an individualized program to achieve and maintain cardiovascular endurance fitness. Because the average American is overfat, Part Three provides assistance in determining how much weight you might need to lose and how to plan a nourishing, well-balanced diet, whether on a weight-loss or weight-maintenance program. Part Four brings together activities combining strength, flexibility, and cardiovascular endurance that can be used at family evenings, family reunions, parties, and for other special events.

Part One

Lift That Barge, Tote That Bale: Muscle Strength and Flexibility

Timmy Livewell, nine, excitedly announced to his family during dinner one evening that he could do more pull-ups and sit-ups than any of his fourth grade classmates. During physical fitness tests in the school gym that day, he had outperformed his peers on those two tests.

Though American children have as many opportunities as children in other countries to engage in vigorous exercise and sports, the average American child is less physically fit than his counterpart in almost any other nation in the Western world. This is no less true of tests to measure muscle strength and flexibility. Pull-ups and sit-ups are measures of strength.

What's so important about strength and flexibility? Aren't they characteristics only the athlete, professional dancer, or man whose work requires hard physical labor cares about? If you think about it, all your daily activities require some degree of strength and flexibility. *Strength* is defined as the ability of the body to exert force against resistance. The greater the resistance, the greater the force required to maintain equilibrium. For instance, maintaining a sitting or standing position requires body force

1

against the resistance of gravity, which tends to pull the body down. It is the muscles of the body that exert this force against resistance. The stronger the muscles, the greater force they can exert against resistance. A mother lifting an infant or child is using strength (force against the resistance of the child's weight). Strength is a prerequisite to any muscle movement and, therefore, necessary to perform any skill. In order to build strength in any given set of muscles, such as the abdominal or lower back muscles which are more often than not weak, exercises requiring progressively more resistance are required.

It is not known what the ideal strength of an adult or child should be. However, you know whether or not you have the strength to do your various day-to-day tasks, such as lifting and carrying children, books, or groceries, pulling a hose from one part of the yard to another, putting stacks of dishes away in the cupboard, shoveling the garden, raking the lawn, pulling open a door that is jammed, pushing a car to get it started, vacuuming the house, moving furniture, and hundreds of other activities.

In any discussion of strength, women tend to "turn off," thinking they will become muscle-bound if they engage in strength-building activities. However, women generally do not have the hormones and genetic blueprints for the development of large and unsightly muscles. A person with adequate strength in his muscles generally has good posture and plenty of vigor and becomes increasingly efficient in daily tasks as well as sports and recreational activities.

Flexibility is also important in any body movement. *Flexibility* is sometimes referred to as the elastic tone of the body — the ability to stretch and bend, to twist and turn without undue stress or pain. It is the ability of any given joint of the body to move through its full range of motion.

Flexibility is specific to a given part of the body. For instance, you can be flexible in the shoulder joints but inflexible in the joints of the lower back or lower limbs. Flexibility problem areas for most Americans are the shoulder girdle and hip extensors. This is probably due to the sedentary life-style of most people, children as well as adults. Inactivity of a muscle leads to loss of its extensibility. Thus, we are unable to move various body parts through their full range of motion.

Stretching is the road to muscle flexibility, just as it is for a rubber band. However, the stretching should be slow and sustained, not fast or jerky or bouncy. Jerking or bouncing a muscle leads to muscle contraction as well as extension, thus counteracting the purpose of the exercise.

During our discussion of strength and flexibility in the two chapters that follow, several words will be used that you should learn now.

Overload principle — constantly working muscles near their limits (gradually increasing duration or frequency of an exercise). As strength

2

increases, the limits also increase, meaning that the body requires more resistance as it exerts an increasingly greater amount of force.

Progressive resistance — gradually increasing the number of repetitions of a given exercise in the same amount of time or gradually increasing the amount of resistance, such as the amount of weight lifted.

Range of motion — the distance a body part can move at a given joint.

Set — a given number of repetitions of an exercise before resting or going on to another exercise.

Repetitions — the number of times a given exercise is repeated.

Resistance — the weight of the body when doing calisthenics or the weight of the dumbbell when weight lifting.

Although ideal flexibility and strength levels are not known, it is still possible to periodically measure your flexibility and strength to see if you are maintaining, increasing, or decreasing either one as you engage in flexibility and strength fitness programs. Therefore, Chapter One describes how to administer and interpret some simple flexibility and strength tests to help you and other family members determine what your starting point is as a means of later comparison.

Chapter Two describes several flexibility and strength exercises that can be done in any home with or without assistance from others. It also describes how to plan and engage in your own individualized flexibility and strength fitness program. The exercises described do not require special equipment usually found in school gymnasiums or expensive health spas. Chapter Two also describes how to engage in your individualized flexibility and strength program. Frequently asked questions about flexibility and strength will be answered and important precautions described.

Chapter One

Appraising Flexibility and Strength

GOAL: Be able to administer and interpret flexibility and strength tests for yourself and any member of your family.

This chapter will help you learn how to administer and interpret four simple flexibility tests and three simple strength tests that can be conducted with equipment generally available in the average household.

The purpose of these tests is to help you and each member of your family determine your own starting point. Fitness levels will not be suggested. As you and members of your family engage in flexibility and strength programs, you can occasionally retake these same tests to find out if you have made any improvements. Remember, you compare yourself with yourself. That is, you compare your later performances on these tests with your starting performance.

PROCEDURES

Each member of the family should fill out a separate flexibility and strength appraisal form as the tests in this chapter are conducted. As these tests are described, notice how nine-year-old Timmy Livewell's form is filled in (Figure 1-1). Timmy's form was filled in when he and the other Livewell family members spent a family evening conducting the test for each other.

If you follow the directions for each of the flexibility and strength tests, you will be able to administer and interpret these tests not only for yourself, but for any other member of your family.

Before beginning the tests, be sure to fill in on line 1 the person's

5

FIGURE 1-1
FLEXIBILITY AND STRENGTH APPRAISAL

1. Name Timmy Livewell _____ Sex M___ Date_____
2. Current body weight_____68 lb._____

Flexibility Tests

3. Hamstring Stretch — Inches_____ Fingers__X___ Joint_____
                     Knuckles_____ Palms_____
4. Tailor Sit Stretch — Inches __6___
5. Shoulder Girdle Rotation — Pass_____ Fail__X___
6. Wing Stretcher — Pass__X___ Fail_____

Strength Tests

7.   a. Modified Pull-ups: arm and shoulder strength. Number of pull-ups before exhaustion_did not take this test_____
     b. Pull-ups: arm and shoulder muscle strength. Number of pull-ups before exhaustion____4____
8. Sit-ups: abdominal and hip muscle strength. Number of complete sit-ups in two minutes__23_____
9.   a. Modified push-ups: forearms, back of upper arms, chest, abdominal muscle strength. Number of push-ups in one minute did not take this test___
     b. Push-ups: forearms, back of upper arms, chest, abdomen muscle strength. Number of push-ups in one minute_____18_____

name, sex, and the date the tests were conducted. The person's weight should be written on line 2.

Flexibility Tests

The flexibility tests do not test all the possible muscle areas of the body. Rather, they are representative tests of muscle flexibility in body areas that are often inflexible.

Hamstring Stretch

Muscles tested: Hamstring muscle group.
Equipment: Yardstick or measuring tape.
Starting position: Person stands erect, shoes off, arms hanging loosely at sides.

Appraising

Action: Lean over and reach finger tips toward the floor without bending knees. Hold position for three seconds as partner measures distance from fingertips to floor or records part of hand that touches the floor.

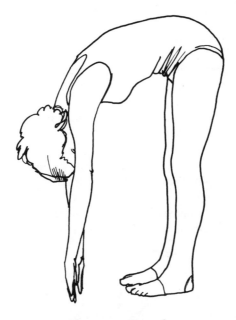

Hamstring Stretch

Rules:
1. The stretching movement should be gradual, not jerky or bouncy.
2. Knees should not bend, neither should they be "locked" into an extended position. They should be straight in line with the ankle bone.
3. Avoid "straining" to touch the floor. This should be a natural, easy movement.
4. The body should remain at full stretch position for the three-second time period.

Scoring: Begin counting time as soon as the person reaches as far as possible without straining or bending knees. If the person is unable to touch the floor with the fingertips, measure the distance from fingertips to the floor and record in inches on line 3. If the person touches the floor with fingertips record fingers on line 3. If the person touches the floor with the first joint of the fingers record joints on line 3. If the person touches the knuckles on the floor record knuckles on line 3. If the person can touch the palms of the hand to the floor record palms on line 3. Timmy Livewell was able to touch his fingertips to the floor so fingers is recorded on line 3 for him.

Tailor Sit Stretch

Muscles tested: Hip extensors.
Equipment: Measuring tape.
Starting position: Sit with soles of feet together, hands grasping toes.
Action: Curl head toward feet while clasping hands over feet.
Rules:
  1. Soles of feet must remain pressed together throughout the test.
  2. Hands remain clasped over feet.
Scoring:
  1. A partner measures the distance from the performer's forehead to the floor. Make sure the measuring instrument is perpendicular (straight line) from forehead to floor.
  2. Record the distance in inches on line 4. Timmy was able to curl his head to within six inches of the floor, so 6 is recorded on line 4.

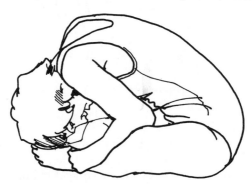

Tailor Sit Stretch

Shoulder Girdle Rotation

Muscles tested: Shoulder girdle.
Equipment: Broomstick or wand thirty-six to forty-two inches long.
Starting position: Stand in a comfortable position gripping broomstick or wand in overhand grip in front of body, one hand near each end, elbows straight.
Action: With elbows straight and firm grip on the broomstick, slowly move the stick over the head and touch it to the lower back.

Appraising

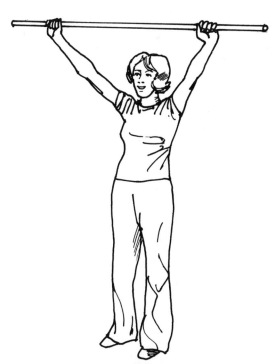

Shoulder Girdle Rotation

Rules:
1. Broomstick must be grasped firmly with overhand grip, one hand at either end.
2. The elbows must remain straight throughout the exercise.
3. Avoid jerky motions.
4. The hands must remain on the broomstick throughout the exercise.

Scoring: This test is recorded either pass or fail. If the performer is able to move the broomstick from front of body to back of body without bending the elbows or releasing the grasp, record a pass. Otherwise, record a fail.

Timmy was not able to keep his elbows straight when he moved the wand over his head. Therefore a fail was recorded on line 5.

Wing Stretcher

Muscles tested: Shoulder girdle.
Equipment: None.

9

Starting position: Normal standing position with arms relaxed at sides of body.

Action: Bring right hand over top of right shoulder to back. At the same time bring left hand under left shoulder to back. Attempt to touch fingers of both hands.

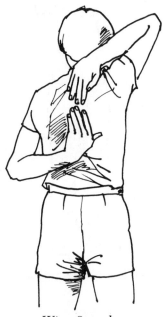

Wing Stretcher

Rules: Bring fingertips together and hold for three seconds.

Scoring: This test is recorded either pass or fail. If the performer is able to touch the fingers of one hand with the fingers of the other hand, record a pass. Otherwise, record a fail.

Timmy was able to touch the fingertips of both hands. Therefore, a pass was recorded on line 6.

Strength Tests

These strength tests do not test all the possible muscle areas of the body. Rather, they are representative tests of body areas that are often weak in muscle strength.

Modified Pull-ups

Muscles tested: Arm and shoulder muscle strength.

Appraising

Equipment: Any bar adjustable in height may be used. The bar should be
comfortable to grip. A piece of pipe placed between two stepladders
and held securely may be used.

Starting position: Adjust height of bar to chest level when the person being
tested is standing. Grasp the bar with palms facing out. Extend legs
under bar keeping body and knees straight. Heels are on floor. Fully
extend arms so they form an angle of 90 degrees with the body line. A
partner braces heels of person being tested to prevent slipping.

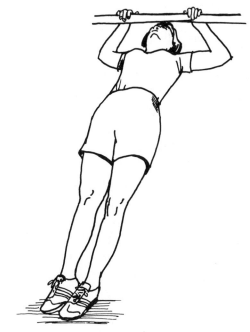

Modified Pull-ups

Action:
1. Pull body up with arms until chest touches the bar.
2. Lower body until elbows are fully extended.
3. Repeat the exercise as many times as possible.

Rules:
1. The body must be kept straight.
2. The chest *must* touch the bar before the arms are then fully
   extended.
3. No resting is permitted.
4. One pull-up is counted each time the chest touches the bar.

11

5.   Continue the exercise as many times as possible without resting.

Scoring: Record the number of completed pull-ups on line 7a for Modified Pull-ups. Partial pull-ups do not count. Timmy Livewell thought he could do the free-hanging pull-ups so he did not take this test.

Pull-ups

Muscles tested: Arm and shoulder muscle strength.

Equipment: A high, horizontal bar or limb of a tree, comfortable to grip.

Starting position: Grasp the bar with palms facing forward, hanging with arms and legs fully extended. Feet must be free of floor or ground. A partner stands slightly to one side of the person being tested and counts each successful pull-up.

Action:

1.   Pull the body up with the arms until chin is raised above bar.

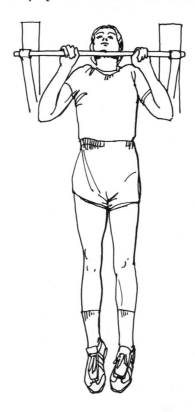

Pull-ups

2. Lower the body until arms are fully extended.
3. Repeat the exercise as many times as possible.

Rules:
1. Avoid pull-ups that are snap movements.
2. Knees must not be raised.
3. Kicking of the legs is not permitted.
4. The body must not swing. If it does, the partner stops the motion by holding an extended arm across the front of the person's thighs.
5. One complete pull-up is counted each time the person places his chin over the bar.
6. Continue the exercise as many times as possible without resting.

Scoring: Record the number of completed pull-ups on line 7. Partial pull-ups do not count. Timmy Livewell completed four pull-ups before exhaustion, so a 4 is recorded on pull-ups line 7b.

Sit-ups

Muscles tested: Abdominal and hip muscle strength.
Equipment: Mat or carpeted floor; stopwatch, watch, or clock with sweep second hand.
Starting position: The person being tested lies on back, knees bent, soles of feet on floor close to buttocks. Hands, with fingers interlocked, are clasped behind neck.

Action:
1. Sit up and turn trunk to the left. Touch right elbow to left knee. Partner begins timing for two minutes as this process begins.
2. Return to starting positon.
3. Sit up and turn trunk to the right, touching left elbow to right knee.

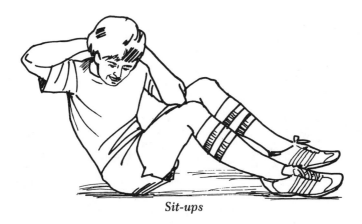

Sit-ups

4. Return to starting position.
5. Do as many sit-ups as possible in two minutes while partner times and counts the sit-ups. Resting between sit-ups is not permitted.
6. One complete sit-up is counted each time the person returns to starting position.

Rules:
1. The fingers must remain in contact behind the neck throughout the exercise.
2. The soles of the feet must remain on the floor during the sit-up. (A partner can hold them down, if necessary.)
3. The back should be rounded and the head and elbows brought forward when sitting up, as a "curl" up.
4. When returning to starting position, elbows must be flat on the mat or floor before sitting up again.

Scoring: One point is given for each complete movement of touching elbow to knee and returning to starting position. No sit-up is counted if fingertips do not maintain contact behind the head, if the feet do not maintain contact with the floor, or if a person pushes up from the floor with an elbow. Allow the person to do as many sit-ups as possible without resting during a *two-minute* interval. Begin timing as soon as the person begins to sit-up from the starting position the first time. Record the number of completed sit-ups in two minutes on line 8. Timmy Livewell was able to complete twenty-three sit-ups in two minutes.

Modified Push-ups

Muscles tested: Forearms, back of upper arms, and chest muscle strength.
Equipment: Mat or carpeted floor; stopwatch, watch, or clock with sweep second hand.

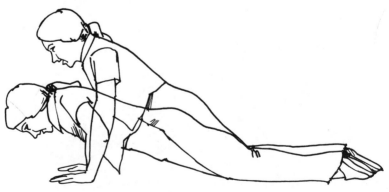

Modified Push-ups

14

Appraising

Starting position: Lie face down on mat or floor, elbows bent, hands placed on floor approximately shoulders' width apart, thumbs next to chest. Partner crouches or kneels nearby to time the person being tested and to count the number of push-ups.

Action:
1. Push body up until arms are straight, with weight of body resting on hands and knees. Keep hips, shoulders, and head all in same straight line.
2. Bend elbows and lower chin to floor.
3. Do as many push-ups as possible in one minute without resting between push-ups.

Rules:
1. Keep hips, shoulders, and head straight during the movement.
2. Do not touch floor with chest.
3. One complete push-up is counted each time the person pushes up to the "straight arm" position and returns to the "chin-on-floor" position. Partial push-ups are not counted.

Scoring: One point is given for each complete push-up. Do not count partial push-ups or those done incorrectly. Allow the person to do as many push-ups as possible without resting during a *one-minute* interval. Begin timing as soon as the person begins the first push-up from the starting position. Record the number of completed push-ups in one minute on line 9a, Modified Push-ups. Timmy knew he could do several full push-ups so he did not take the modified push-up test.

Push-ups

Muscles tested: Forearms, back of upper arms, and chest muscle strength.
Equipment: Mat or carpeted floor; stopwatch, watch, or clock with sweep second hand.
Starting position: Lie face down on mat or floor, elbows bent, hands placed on floor, thumbs next to chest. Partner crouches or kneels nearby to time person being tested and to count the number of push-ups.

Action:
1. Push body up until arms are straight, with weight of body resting on hands and toes, keeping heels, hips, shoulders, and head all in the same straight line.
2. Bend elbows and lower chin to floor.
3. Do as many push-ups as possible in one minute without resting between push-ups.

Rules:
1. Keep body line straight during movement.

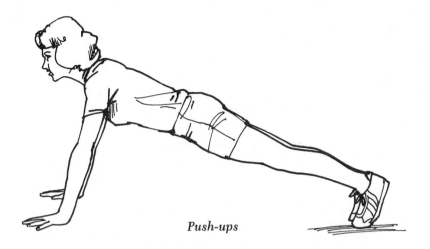

Push-ups

2.   Do not touch floor with chest.
3.   One complete push-up is counted each time the person pushes up to "straight arm" position then returns to starting position. Partial push-ups are not counted.

Scoring: One point is given for each completed push-up. No push-up is counted if body line is not kept straight or if the person touches floor with chest. Allow the person to do as many push-ups as possible without resting during a *one-minute* interval. Begin timing as soon as the person begins the first push-up from the starting position. Record the number of completed push-ups in one minute on line 9b, Push-ups. Timmy Livewell took this test and completed eighteen push-ups in one minute.

Chapter Two

Planning a Flexibility and Strength Fitness Program

GOAL: Be able to achieve and maintain the good or excellent level of fitness by engaging in your own personalized flexibility and strength fitness program.

Chapter 1 helped you appraise your present level of flexibility and strength for representative muscles of your body. The results of these tests will be useful in planning your own fitness program and should be retained for comparison when you repeat the tests every four to six weeks as you participate in the program.

This chapter explains the principles of conditioning that should be followed for consistent and effective results. It also describes five series of flexibility and strength exercises, grouped according to level of difficulty. Each series includes exercises to increase the flexibility and strength of each muscle group in your body.

Series I is the Starter Program, designed to tone each part of the body to minimize the possibility of stiff and sore muscles. The Starter Program will also help you identify the areas of your body that need special attention for fitness conditioning.

The exercises in Series II are progressively more difficult than Series I and, if performed correctly, will bring about a minimal level of fitness and prepare the body to engage in Series III exercises. Series III exercises will help you achieve an average fitness level. After performing Series III exercises for four to six weeks, you will be ready to begin Series IV.

Series IV exercises will help you achieve the good category of physical fitness. With this level of fitness, you are able to engage in regular daily

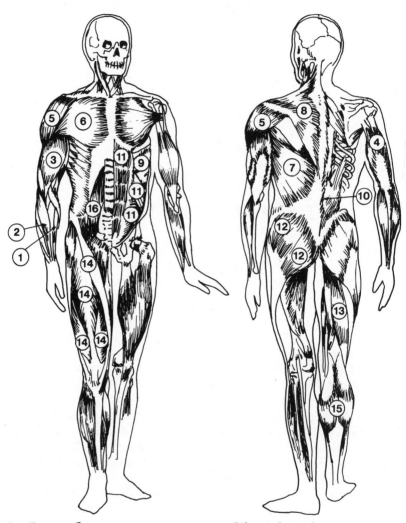

1. Forearm flexors
2. Brachioradialis
3. Biceps
4. Triceps
5. Deltoid
6. Pectoral muscles
7. Latissimus dorsi
8. Trapezius
9. Serratus anterior
10. Erector spinae
    (spinal extensors)
11. Abdominal muscles
    a. Internal and external
       obliques
    b. Rectus abdominus
    c. Transversalis
12. Gluteal muscles
13. Hamstrings
14. Quadriceps muscles
15. Gastrocnemius, soleus muscles
16. Iliopsoas (under abdominal muscles)

activities, recreation, sports, and dance with vitality and freedom from strain to the body. Series V exercises are designed for the person who wants to condition for strenuous physical activity, such as competitive sports, dance performances, etc.

The Jump Rope, Broomstick, and other Family Challenge series in Part Four are designed to add variety and motivation for your fitness pleasure. These series may be substituted into your personal weekly program when desired and may be used for special family and neighborhood occasions.

The accompanying model of the skeletal muscles will help you identify muscle groups and become aware of their functions as you engage in exercises to attain total body conditioning. Generally, activities that extend or stretch the muscles increase flexibility, and activities that shorten or contract the muscles increase strength. As you engage in fitness activities, become better acquainted with your own muscular system and what takes place when the muscles are contracted and extended.

PRINCIPLES OF CONDITIONING

To attain the full benefits of your fitness program, you should understand and practice the following principles: The body is designed for activity; it is strengthened by use and becomes weak when not used. When a person's body is conditioned by a sequentially planned program of progressive resistance exercises, he or she will be able to perform daily tasks with ease and have a strength and energy reserve for recreational pursuits or unexpected events.

We are surrounded by people who are exhausted at the end, or even midway through, their day, as a result of physical exertion. However, they do not reach a higher level of conditioning due to the inconsistency and lack of progression of activities in which they are engaged.

Progressive resistance is defined as a gradual increase in the number of repetitions in the same amount of time or a gradual increase in the resistance applied. To understand how this principle works in your personal fitness program, let's review the series of exercises in this chapter.

First, you will note that for each exercise, the number of times the exercise should be performed is shown: Head Rotation — 4-8 means that the head rotation should be performed four times the first day and increased by one or two additional times until you are performing it eight times. Repeat this number four or five exercise periods before moving to the next series. The directions for head rotation state that you should rotate the head by making large circles with the nose, trying to increase the size of the circles each exercise period. By keeping the body stationary as the head is rotated in large circles, a progressive resistance is realized. In most exercises, the body position provides the resistance; as the body becomes stronger, it provides a greater amount of resistance. You will note that additional weight is added when performing some exercises. The resistance is increased in the arm circles in Series II by holding an empty bottle in each hand and in Series III adding additional weight by using bottles that are full. Perform each exercise as directed to realize the full benefits of progressive resistance.

Intensity

Intensity is defined as the energy demands placed upon the body for any given exercise. Begin slowly and progress cautiously to find the level at which you can exercise for the best conditioning. If you begin at too high a level, you will become exhausted and unable to complete your program. However, if you do not work or place demands upon the muscles, they will not increase in flexibility or strength, and you will become discouraged. Remember, the words of caution are *begin slowly* and *progress*, exerting a little more energy each exercise period. Do not compete with other members of the family or friends, but progress at your own level.

Frequency

Research studies have found that the body begins to lose its ability to perform at the same level as few as twenty-four hours after the level has been achieved. We are also told that in order to receive continuing fitness benefits, we must repeat the activity within every forty-eight hours. This information directs us to schedule a daily or at least every-other-day program for fitness. Some family groups exercise together early in the morning, others find it more convenient to exercise before retiring at night. The time of day is not important; however, the regularity and consistency of the exercise period is of utmost importance.

The sequence in which the exercises are performed will add to the effectiveness of the program. Stretching exercises bring about flexibility and warm-up or tone the muscle groups for more demanding strength exercises. At the conclusion of the flexibility and strength series, the body is warmed-up and ready for aerobic activity. At the conclusion of the aerobic activity, it is important to have a five- to ten-minute period of cooling-down activity to gradually bring the body functions back to normal.

PROCEDURES

Read the directions for the exercise described in the Starter Program (Series I). If you have been sedentary for a period of time, you should start the program by performing the lowest number of repetitions. If you have been fairly active and were able to pass the flexibility and strength tests, perform each exercise at the higher number of repetitions.

✓ It is important that all flexibility exercises be performed with a sustained, controlled stretch. *Do not bounce or bob* on stretched muscles. This is not only ineffective for attaining flexibility, but also causes stiffness and possible pulling of muscle tissues.

✓ The program has been designed to allow you to attain physical fitness without the discomfort of stiff and sore muscles. It is important that you begin the program slowly — to allow your body to adjust to the stress of additional activity — and then progress according to the recommended number of repetitions in each series before moving to the next series.

With information you learned about your present condition from the flexibility and strength tests and that which you learned by reviewing the Starter Program, you are ready to chart your personal fitness program.

The Livewell family charted their programs the same evening they helped each other with the flexibility and strength tests. Sharon Livewell didn't do very well on the flexibility and strength tests, so she started Series I exercises at the lowest number of repetitions. Tina passed all the flexibility tests, so she performed Series I exercises at the highest number of repetitions. However, she didn't do very well on the strength tests, so she started Series I strength exercises at the lowest number of repetitions.

Jon did very well on the strength tests but was poor in flexibility. He decided this was the reason he had stiff, sore muscles after going on a mountain-climbing outing. Jon's personal fitness program started with flexibility exercises in Series I, strength exercises for push-ups and pull-ups in Series III, and all other strength exercises in Series II. Tina and Michelle were both high in flexibility and low in strength, so they decided to follow the same program. That way, Michelle could watch Tina and learn how to do the exercises.

Chart your own personal fitness program by writing the date (month and day) in the space provided by each exercise. Each time you have performed the highest number of repetitions in one series for at least a week and feel you are ready to progress to the next series, you will write the date you start the new series by that particular exercise.

SERIES I

Flexibility

I-1. Head Rotation

Starting position: Sit or stand erect.

FIGURE 2-1
INDIVIDUAL FITNESS PROGRESS CHART

Body Area Conditioned	Starter Program Series I	Rep.	Date	Series II	Rep.	Date
Neck Hands Wrist	*Flexibility* 1. Head Rotation 2. Finger Flex	4-8 10-15		*Flexibility* 1. Head Rotation 2. Wrist Flex	8-10 4-8	
Arms Shoulders	3. Arm Rotation 1 4. Wing Stretcher 1	10-15 4-8		3. Arm Rotation 2 4. Wing Stretcher 2	10-15 4-8	
Mid-body Waist	5. Side Bender 6. Toe Toucher 1	1-4 4-8		5. Body Bender 6. Torso Twist	1-4 4-8	
Back	7. Hamstring Stretch 1	4-8		7. Hamstring Stretch 2	4-8	
Hamstrings Hips	8. Low Back Stretch 1 9. Nose to Knees 1	4-8 4-8		8. Low Back Stretch 1 9. Nose to Knees 1	8-10 10-15	
				10. Nose to Knees 2	4-8	
				11. Sitting Stride Stretch	4-8	
	10. Tailor Sit 1	4-8		12. Tailor Sit 2	4-8	
Legs Feet	11. Foot Rotation 12. Heel Cord Stretch 1	4-8 6-8		13. Foot Rotation 14. Heel Cord Stretch 1	8-10 6-8	
Neck	*Strength* 13. Head Resist	4-8		*Strength* 15. Head Pull	4-8	
Hands Arms Shoulders Chest	14. Hand Clencher 15. Hand Pull 16. Arm Raise 1 17. Modified Push-ups 1	4-8 4-8 4-8 3-10		16. Ball Squeeze 17. Hand Pull 18. Arm Raise 2 19. Elbow Raise 20. Modified Push-ups 2	4-8 8-12 4-8 4-8 10-35	
Back Abdomen Hips Buttocks	18. Chest Raiser 1 19. Angry Cat 20. Abdominal Curls 1 21. Side Leg Lift 1	4-8 4-8 4-12 4-8		21. Chest Raiser 1 22. Angry Cat 23. Abdominal Curls 1 24. Leg Raiser 1 25. Side Leg Lift 1	8-10 8-10 12-30 3-6 8-15	
Legs Feet	22. Toe Walk 23. Arch Strengthener	10-20 5-10		26. Step-Knee Touch 27. Toe to Heel Rock	4-8 4-8	
	Cardiovascular *Endurance* Vigorous walk, swim, or cycle	5-15 minutes		*Cardiovascular* *Endurance* Walk-jog, dance, swim or cycle within conditioning zone	1-1½ miles 15-20 minutes	

FIGURE 2-1
INDIVIDUAL FITNESS PROGRESS CHART

Series III	Rep.	Date	Series IV	Rep.	Date	Series V	Rep.	Date
Flexibility			*Flexibility*			*Flexibility*		
1. Head Rotation	10		1. Head Rotation	10		1. Head Lift	8-15	
2. Hand Rotation	4-8		2. Hand Rotation	8				
3. Wrist Backbend	4-8		3. Wrist Backbend	8				
4. Arm Rotation 3	8-20		4. Arm Circles 1	15-20		2. Arm Circles 2	15-25	
5. Wing Stretcher 3	4-8		5. Wing Stretcher 3	8-12				
6. Body Bender	4-6		6. Body Bender	6		3. Body Bender	4-6	
7. Toe Toucher 2	4-8		7. Hamstring Stretch 3	4-8		4. Hamstring Stretch 4	4-8	
8. Low Back Stretch 1	10		8. Low Back Stretch 1	10		5. Hamstring Stretch 5	4-8	
9. Low Back Stretch 2	4-8		9. Low Back Stretch 2	8		6. Seated Leg Lift	8-12	
10. Nose to Knees 1	15		10. Nose to Knees 1	15		7. Sitting Stride Stretch 2	8-12	
11. Nose to Knees 2	10-15		11. Nose to Knees 2	15		8. Sitting Stride Stretch 3	25	
12. Sitting Stride Stretch	10-15		12. Sitting Stride Stretch	15-20		9. Tailor Sit 4	8-12	
13. Tailor Sit 3	4-8		13. Tailor Sit 3	8-12		10. Hurdle Stretch	10	
14. 3 Count Leg Swing	4-6		14. Hurdle Stretch	4-8		11. Low Back Stretch 3	4-8	
15. Heel Cord Stretch 1	8-10		15. Heel Cord Stretch 1	8		12. High Kicks	20-30	
16. Heel Cord Stretch 2	4-8		16. Heel Cord Stretch 2	8		13. Heel Cord Stretch 1	8	
						14. Heel Cord Stretch 2	8	
Strength			*Strength*			*Strength*		
17. Head Pull	8-12		17. Head Pull	12		15. Head Pull	15	
18. Modified Pull-ups	4-10		18. Pull-ups	2-6		16. Pull-ups	6-10	
19. Arm Raise 3	4-8							
20. Elbow Raise	8-10							
21. Push-ups	4-15		19. Push-ups	15-25		17. Push-ups	25-50	
22. Chest Raiser 2	6-10		20. Chest Raiser 2	10-15		18. Abdominal Curls 3	30-50	
23. Abdominal Curls 2	12-30		21. Abdominal Curls 3	12-30		19. Abdominal Curls 4	15-25	
24. Leg Raiser 2	3-6		22. Leg Raiser 2	6-10		20. V Curl-ups	10-20	
25. Side Leg Lift 2	6-10		23. Side Leg Lift 2	10-15		21. Back Leg Lift	10-20	
26. Step-Knee Touch	9-15		24. Knee Bends	10-20		22. Knee Bends	25	
27. Wall Sit	1 min.		25. Wall Sit	2 min.		23. Ankle Bounce	20-30	
28. Toe to Heel Rock	8-12		26. Ankle Bounce	20-30		24. Tuck Jumping	15-25	
Cardiovascular Endurance			*Cardiovascular Endurance*			*Cardiovascular Endurance*		
Jog, dance, jumprope, swim or cycle within conditioning zone	1½-2 miles 20-25 min.		Jog, swim, dance, jumprope or cycle within conditioning zone	20-30 min.		Jog, swim, dance, cycle or jumprope within conditioning zone	30-40 min.	

23

Action: Rotate head by making large circular motions with nose. Try to increase size of circle each exercise period. Begin with 4 rotations clockwise, repeat with 4 rotations counterclockwise. Gradually increase the number of rotations to 8 in each direction.

I-2. Finger Flex

Action: This exercise is performed by alternately clenching fists and then extending fingers forcefully. Repeat 10 times, gradually working to 15.

I-3. Arm Rotation 1

Starting position: Sit or stand erect, arms held out to sides shoulder height, palms up.

Action: Contract shoulder blades together, rotate the arms in small circles with a backward rotation (clockwise). Begin with 10 rotations, gradually increasing to 15.

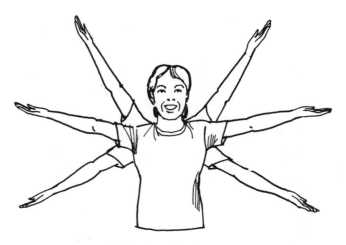

I-3.   Arm Rotation

I-4. Wing Stretcher 1

Starting position: Stand erect, arms bent at elbows, hands held shoulder high, fingers touching, palms down.

Action: Pull elbows back as far as possible, keeping hands and arms shoulder height. Pull back on count one, return to starting position on count two. Begin with 4 and gradually increase to 8.

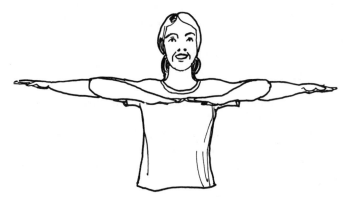

I-4. Wing Stretcher 1

I-5. Side Bender

Starting position: Stand in comfortable side stride position, feet approximately eighteen inches apart.

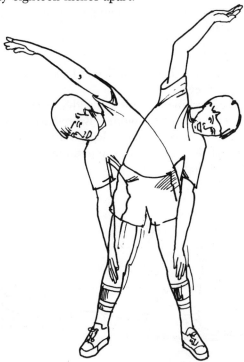

I-5. Side Bender

Action: Bring right arm over head, reach to left with entire upper body. At the same time reach left hand down left side, gently stretch, for a count of 8 to the left. Change positions and repeat to right. Gradually work to 4 sets of 8 on each side.

I-6. Toe Toucher 1

Starting position: Stand in wide stride position, arms outstretched to sides shoulder height.

Action: Bend forward, bringing right hand toward left toe. Come to an upright position and repeat, bringing left hand toward right toe. Repeat at a rapid pace 4 times, gradually increasing to 8 times on each side.

I-7. Hamstring Stretch 1

Starting position: Stand erect, feet together.

Action: Slowly bend body forward, *keeping knees straight* (with straight line through center of knees to ankle bone). Reach hands toward floor. *Do not* bob or bounce in this position. Hold in extended position for count of three, return to standing position. Repeat 4 times, gradually working to 8.

I-8. Low Back Stretch 1

Starting position: Lie on back, bend right leg at knee, at the same time forcefully extend left leg.

Action: Grasp right knee with both hands and with a smooth, continuous motion, pull knee toward right shoulder. Extend arms back to original position. Repeat 3 times. Change leg positions and repeat the same action with left leg. Start with 4 repetitions and gradually increase to 8 with each leg.

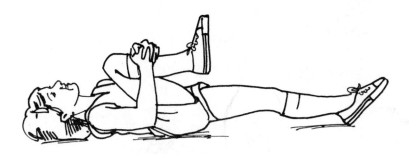

I-8. Low Back Stretch 1

I-9. Nose to Knees 1

Starting position: Sit erect on floor, legs extended, back straight, ankles extended.

Action: Reach fingers toward toes, *keeping knees straight,* and curl head toward knees. Action should be a smooth continuous stretch forward. Repeat 4 times, gradually working to 8.

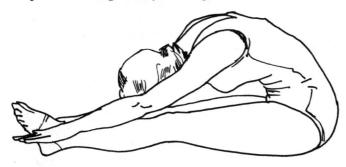

I-9.   *Nose to Knees 1*

I-10. Tailor Sit 1

Starting position: Sit on floor, soles of feet together, grasping feet with both hands.

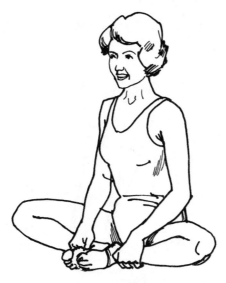

I-10.   *Tailor Sit 1*

Action: Gently pull feet closer to buttocks. Repeat 4 times, trying to get feet closer to body each time. Gradually work to 8 repetitions.

I-11. Foot Rotation

Starting position: Sitting on chair.

Action: From sitting position on a chair, extend one leg forward. Hold upper part of leg still and rotate foot at ankle by drawing large circles in the air with toes. Make circles in a clockwise direction 4 times. Repeat in counterclockwise direction. Repeat with other leg. Gradually work to 8 repetitions.

I-12. Heel Cord Stretch 1

Starting position: Stand facing a wall or solid surface with feet fifteen to eighteen inches from wall. Place hands on body in straight alignment from heels through head.

Action: Lean to the wall. At the same time push down on heels, to keep them flat against floor. Push back to straight standing position to repeat exercise. Move feet farther from the wall as flexibility increases. Repeat 6-8 times each day, gradually moving feet a greater distance from the wall.

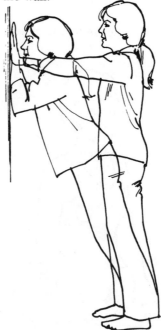

I-12.   Heel Cord Stretch 1

Strength

I-13. Head Resist

Starting position: Sit or stand, back erect, hands clasped behind head, elbows level with hands.

Action: Press forward with hands, at the same time resisting with head by maintaining a rigid position with neck for a four-second count. Repeat 4 times, gradually working to 8.

I-14. Hand Clencher

Starting position: Sit or stand, hands in clenched fist position.

Action: Alternately squeeze and relax hands. Start with 4 repetitions and gradually work to 8.

I-15. Hand Pull

Starting position: Sit or stand, hands and elbows raised to shoulder level, fingers curled.

Action: Overlap fingers and pull through hands and shoulders. Hold for a four-second count and then relax for a two-second count. Start with 4 repetitions and gradually work to 8.

I-16. Arm Raise 1

Starting position: Lie face down on floor, arms stretched to sides shoulder height.

Action: Raise arms off floor for a four-second count. Return to starting position. Repeat. Keep arms at shoulder height throughout exercise. Start with 4 and gradually work to 8.

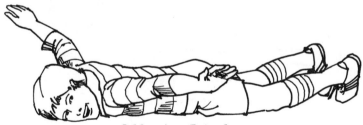

I-16. Arm Raise 1

I-17. Modified Push-ups 1

Starting position: Kneel on hands and knees, hands directly under shoulders.

Action: Lower body until chin touches floor. Return to starting position. Repeat as many times as possible each exercise period. When you are able to do 10 push-ups, increase the distance between hands and knees until your body is in a straight line from knees to shoulders.

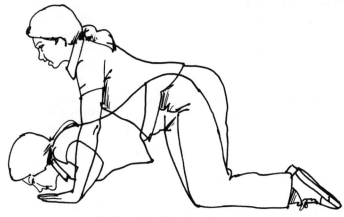

I-17.   Modified Push-ups 1

I-18. Chest Raiser 1

Starting position: Lie face down on floor, hands clasped in middle of back.
Action: Leading with the chin, raise shoulders off floor as high as possible. Hold for a four-second count, return to starting position. Start with 4 repetitions and gradually increase to 8.

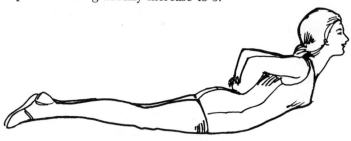

I-18.   Chest Raiser 1

I-19. Angry Cat

Starting position: Support body on hands and knees (shoulders' width apart). Head and buttocks are raised and back is lowered (like a broken-down horse).

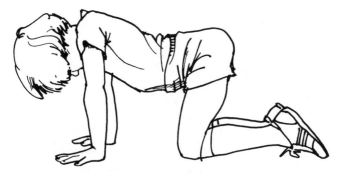

I-19. Angry Cat
(Starting position)

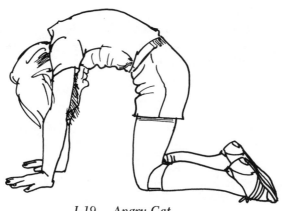

I-19. Angry Cat
(Action)

Action: Contract belly muscles forming an arch with back. Lower head and buttocks for a four-second count. Return to starting position. Start with 4 repetitions, gradually increasing to 8.

I-20. Abdominal Curls 1

Starting position: Lie on back, knees bent, feet on floor, heels close to buttocks, arms outstretched toward knees.
Action: Slowly curl head and shoulders forward, reaching fingers toward knees. The curl should be slow and smooth. At the same time flatten belly muscles with a pull toward the back. Curl forward for a two-second count. Return to starting position. Begin with 4 repetitions and gradually increase to 12.

31

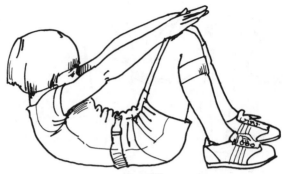

I-20.   Abdominal Curls 1

I-21. Side Leg Lift 1

Starting position: Lie on right side, body in straight line, right arm extended under head. Place left hand in front of body to help maintain this position throughout exercise.

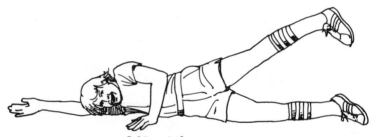

I-21.   Side Leg Lift 1

Action: Raise left leg upward, leading with heel on count one, lowering on count two. Repeat 4 times on each side, gradually increasing to 8.

I-22. Toe Walk

Starting position: Stand erect, balancing weight on balls of feet.
Action: Walk forward, maintaining weight on balls of feet for 10 steps on each foot, gradually increasing to 20.

I-23. Arch Strengthener

Starting position: Sit erect.
Action: Curl toes under feet for a four-second count. Relax. Repeat. Pick up small objects such as marbles, chalk, etc., by curling toes around them. Move objects from one place to another. Repeat 5-10 times.

SERIES II

Flexibility

II-1. Head Rotation

Do this exercise as described in Series I-1. Repeat 8-10 times.

II-2. Wrist Flex

Starting position: Sitting or standing.
Action: Gently push thumb of left hand toward left forearm. Repeat by gently pushing right thumb toward right forearm. Do 4-8 times for each hand.

II-3. Arm Rotation 2

Starting position: Stand erect, arms extended sideward shoulder height, palms up, grasping an empty pop bottle in each hand.
Action: Rotate arms in small circles with a backward turning motion. 10-15 times.

II-4. Wing Stretcher 2

Starting position: Sit or stand erect.
Action: Bring right hand over top of right shoulder to back. At the same time bring left hand under shoulder to back. Stretch hands toward

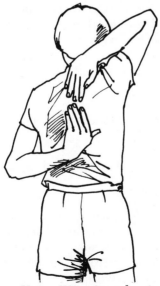

II-4. Wing Stretcher 2

each other, attempting to touch finger tips. Do 4 times on each side, attempting to increase the grasp each time. Gradually increase to 8 repetitions on each side.

II-5. Body Bender

Starting position: Stand erect, feet shoulder width apart.
Action:

1. Extend right arm over head and reach to left with entire upper body, at the same time reaching left hand down left side as far as possible. Gently stretch for eight consecutive counts.
2. Place hands on hips, extend chin, lean back. Gently stretch for eight consecutive counts.
3. Repeat action 1 to the opposite side. (Completion of 1, 2, 3 above comprises one set.) Begin with 1 set, gradually increasing to 4 sets.

II-6. Torso Twist

Starting position: Stand erect, hands on hips, feet shoulder width apart.
Action: Rotate upper body to right, at the same time resist with lower body. Repeat to left. Start with 4 repetitions and gradually work to 8.

II-7. Hamstring Stretch 2

Starting position: Stand erect, feet together.
Action: With slow sustained stretch, bend body forward, extending palms of hands toward floor. Stretch forward on count one and two, hold stretched position for count three, return to starting position on count four. Keep knees straight for the four-second count. Start with 4 repetitions and gradually work to 8.

II-8. Low Back Stretch 1

Do this exercise as described in Series I-8. Repeat 8-10 times with each leg.

II-9. Nose to Knees 1

Do this exercise as described in Series I-9. Repeat 10-15 times.

II-10. Nose to Knees 2

Starting position: Sit on floor, feet extended, toes flexed toward knees.
Action: Curl head toward knees. Keep knees straight and toes flexed toward knees. Stretch hands toward toes and head toward knees with a slow, sustained four-second count. Stretch forward, returning to starting position. Repeat 4-8 times.

34

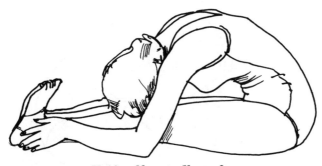

II-10.   Nose to Knees 2

II-11. Sitting Stride Stretch 1

Starting position: Sit erect on floor, legs in wide stride position.
Action: With a smooth sustained stretch, bend upper body forward, reaching hands to floor in center of body. On a four-second count, reach forward and then return to starting position. Repeat 4-8 times.

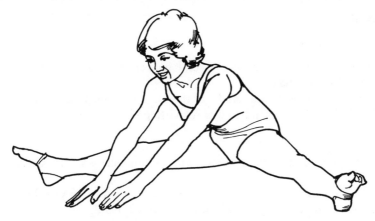

II-11.   Sitting Stride Stretch 1

II-12. Tailor Sit 2

Starting position: Sit on floor, soles of feet together, grasp feet with both hands.
Action: Gently pull feet toward body to a position in line with knees, at the same time gently curl head toward feet for a four-second count. Return to starting position. Repeat 4-8 times.

35

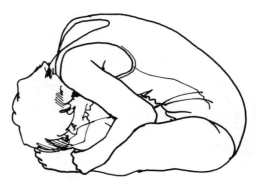

II-12.   Tailor Sit 2

II-13. Foot Rotation

Do this exercise as described in Series I-11. Repeat 8-10 times.

II-14. Heel Cord Stretch 1

Do this exercise as described in Series I-12. Repeat 6-8 times.

Strength

II-15. Head Pull

Starting Position: Sit with back erect, hands clasped behind head, elbows
  level with hands.
Action: Pull forward with hands, at the same time push back with head.
  Pull for a four-second count, relax. Repeat 4-8 times.

II-16. Ball Squeeze

Starting position: Sit or stand erect with a tennis ball (or similar size) in left
  hand.
Action: Squeeze the ball, exerting as much pressure as possible for a
  four-second count. Do 4-8 times with each hand.

II-17. Hand Pull

Do this exercise as described in Series I-15. Repeat 8-12 times.

II-18. Arm Raise 2

Starting position: Lie face down on floor, head turned to side, arms
  extended above head at 45-degree angle from shoulders.
Action: Raise arms off floor for a four-second count. Return to starting
  position (try to maintain the 45-degree angle throughout the exercise).
  Repeat 4-8 times.

II-19. Elbow Raise

Starting position: Lie face down on floor, head turned to side, elbows brought to a 90-degree angle shoulder height.

Action: While maintaining 90-degree angle at the elbow, bring shoulder blades together and raise hands, arms, and elbows (as a unit) off the floor. All other parts of body remain on floor. Hold for a four-second count. Return to starting position. Repeat 4-8 times.

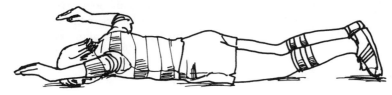

II-19.   Elbow Raise

II-20. Modified Push-ups 2

Starting position: Lie face down on floor with hands directly under shoulders, fingers pointing forward.

Action: Push off floor until arms are fully extended and body is supported by hands and knees. Body should be in a straight line from head to knees. Lower body until chin touches floor on count one, on count two raise body to full arm extension. Repeat 10-35 times.

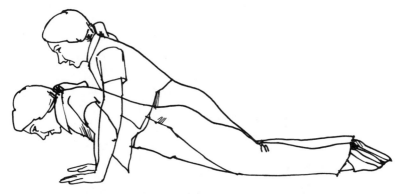

II-20.   Modified Push-ups 2

II-21. Chest Raiser 1

Do this exercise as described in Series I-18. Repeat 8-10 times.

II-22. Angry Cat

Do this exercise as described in Series I-19. Repeat 8-10 times.

II-23. Abdominal Curls 1

Do this exercise as described in Series I-20. Repeat 12-30 times.

II-24. Leg Raiser 1

Starting position: Lie on floor, face resting on hands, legs extended.
Action: Maintain both hip bones on floor and raise left leg in the air to a slow count of four. Return to starting position and repeat with right leg. Do 3-6 for each leg.

II-25. Side Leg Lift 1

Do this exercise as described in Series I-21. Repeat 8-15 times.

II-26. Step-Knee Touch

Starting position: Stand erect, arms out to sides for balance.
Action: Step forward on right foot. While maintaining weight on right foot, touch left knee to floor. Return to starting position. Repeat by stepping with left foot. Do 4-8 times on each leg.

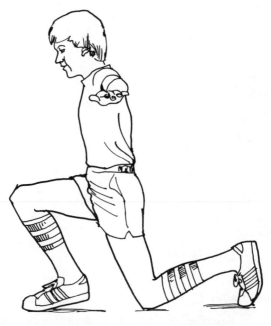

II-26.   Step-Knee Touch

II-27. Toe to Heel Rock

Starting position: Stand erect, hands out to sides, weight balanced on balls of feet.
Action: Rock on outer borders of feet from balls to heels. Return to starting position. Repeat 4-8 times.

SERIES III

Flexibility

III-1. Head Rotation

Do this exercise as described in Series I-1. Repeat 10 times.

III-2. Hand Rotation

Starting position: Stand or sit erect.
Action: Rotate hands at wrist in large circles clockwise. Repeat counterclockwise. Make 4-8 circles in each direction.

III-3. Wrist Backbend

Starting position: Stand or sit erect.
Action: Hold right hand in front of right shoulder, palm forward. With left hand, gently pull right hand backward. Repeat with opposite hand. Do 4-8 times with each hand.

III-4. Arm Rotation 3

Starting position: Stand erect, arms extended sideward, palms up, grasping a filled pop bottle in each hand.
Action: Contract shoulder blades and maintain this position as you rotate arms in small circles in a backward turning motion. Make 8-20 rotations.

III-5. Wing Stretcher 3

Starting position: Stand erect, feet in forward stride position with a rope held taut in front of body (a rod, towel, broomstick, etc., approximately thirty-six inches long can be used).
Action: Raise arms as high as possible over head and back without bending elbows, at the same time keep rope taut. Each day attempt to extend the rope farther back until you can touch it to your back without bending elbows. Return to starting position. Repeat 4-8 times.

III-6. Body Bender

Do this exercise as described in Series II-5. Start with 4 sets and increase to 6 sets.

III-7. Toe Toucher 2

Starting position: Stand in wide stride position, feet approximately two feet apart, arms extended, hands clasped overhead.

Action: Bend the body forward, reaching hands toward right toes. Return to starting position and repeat by reaching toward left toes. The action should be a slow, sustained stretch. Repeat 4-8 times.

III-8. Low Back Stretch 1

Do this exercise as described in Series I-8. Repeat 10 times with each leg.

III-9 Low Back Stretch 2

Starting position: Lie on back, bend knees and grasp one knee with each hand, holding each knee in line with each shoulder.

Action: Pull both knees at the same time toward the respective shoulder. Hold for a four-second count and return to starting position. Repeat 4-8 times.

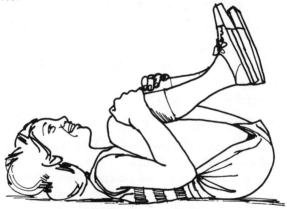

III-9.   Low Back Stretch 2

III-10. Nose to Knees 1

Do this exercise as described in Series I-9. Repeat 15 times.

III-11. Nose to Knees 2

Do this exercise as described in Series II-10. Repeat 10-15 times.

III-12. Sitting Stride Stretch

Do this exercise as described in Series II-11. Progress by reaching farther forward, lowering head closer to the floor and extending legs farther apart. Repeat 10-15 times.

III-13. Tailor Sit 3

Starting position: Sit on floor, soles of feet together, grasping feet with both
hands, bringing them to a position in line with knees.

Action: Push knees down toward floor with elbows. At the same time gently
curl head toward feet for a four-second count. Return to starting
position. Repeat 4-8 times.

III-14. Three Count Leg Swing

Starting position: Stand erect, side toward wall. Hold chair or solid object
to maintain balance.

Action: Maintain weight on left leg, keep upper torso erect, rotate right leg
out and swing it forward on count 1 (return to starting position),
sideward on count 2 (return to starting position), and backward on
count 3 (return to starting position). This sequence completes one set.
Do 4-6 sets.

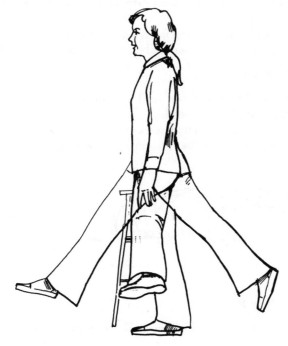

III-14.   Three Count Leg Swing

III-15. Heel Cord Stretch 1

Do this exercise as described in Series I-12. Repeat 8-10 times.

III-16. Heel Cord Stretch 2

Starting position: Stand in forward stride position, hands extended in front of shoulders against wall, forward leg bent with foot approximately eighteen inches from wall, back leg extended, heel flat against floor.

Action: Lean body to touch chin to wall, keeping a straight line from head to heel. Press heel of back leg to floor for a four-second count. Change feet and repeat. Do 4-8 times for each leg.

Strength

III-17. Head Pull

Do this exercise as described in Series II-15. Repeat 8-12 times.

III-18. Modified Pull-ups

Equipment needed: Securely fastened overhead rope or horizontal bar.

Starting position: Lie on back, arms extended to bar. Grasp bar, fingers curled forward.

Action: With only heels touching floor, raise body to bring chin over bar. Repeat 4-10 times, maintaining body weight on heels and hands.

III-19. Arm Raise 3

Starting position: Lie face down on floor, head turned to side, arms extended straight above head.

Action: Lift arms off floor for a four-second count, at the same time keep all other body parts on the floor. Return to starting position. Repeat 4-8 times.

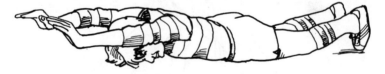

III-19.   Arm Raise 3

III-20. Elbow Raise

Do this exercise as described in Series II-19. Repeat 8-10 times.

III-21. Push-ups

Starting position: Lie face down on floor, palms on floor under shoulders, fingers pointed forward, legs extended.

Action: With arms extended, maintain body weight on hands and toes.

Keep body in a straight line from head to toes. Lower chin to floor by bending arms. Repeat as many times as possible, gradually increasing to 15.

III-22. Chest Raiser 2

Starting position: Lie face down on floor, hands clasped behind head.
Action: Lead with the head in raising upper body off floor as far as possible. Hold for a count of two, return to starting position. Repeat 6-10 times.

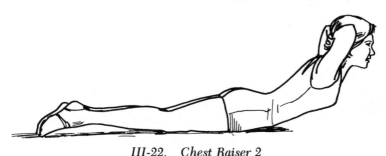

III-22.   Chest Raiser 2

III-23. Abdominal Curls 2

Starting position: Lie on back, knees bent, feet on floor, heels close to buttocks, arms folded across chest.
Action: Slowly curl head and shoulders forward for a two-second count. Touch elbows to knees. Return to starting position for a two-second count. Repeat 12-30 times.

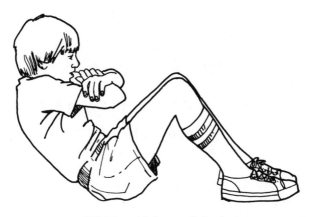

III-23.   Abdominal Curls 2

III-24. Leg Raiser 2

Starting position: Lie on floor, face resting on hands, left leg extended, right leg bent with toes pointing toward ceiling.

Action: Keeping *both hip bones* on floor, raise right leg for a four-second count. Return to starting position. Repeat 3-6 times. Repeat with left leg.

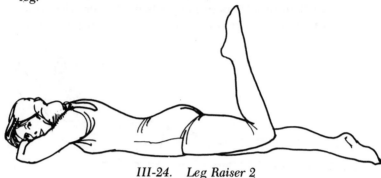

III-24.   Leg Raiser 2

III-25. Side Leg Lift 2

Starting position: Lie on right side, body in straight line, right arm extended under head, left arm in front of body for support.

Action: Raise left leg upward, leading with heel. Hold for a count of two. Bring right leg up to touch left leg. Hold for a count of two. Lower both legs. Repeat 6-10 times. Lie on left side and repeat.

III-26. Step-Knee Touch

Do this exercise as described in Series II-26. Do 9-15 steps on each leg.

III-27. Wall Sit

Starting Position: Stand with back against wall, knees bent to a 90-degree angle, feet flat on floor.

Action: Hold this position for a four-second count. Gradually increase the amount of time you can hold this position to one minute.

III-28. Toe to Heel Rock

Do this exercise as described in Series II-27. Repeat 8-12 times.

SERIES IV
Maintenance Level

Flexibility

IV-1. Head Rotation

Do this exercise as described in Series I-1. Repeat 10 times.

IV-2. Hand Rotation

Do this exercise as described in Series III-2. Repeat 8 times.

IV-3. Wrist Backbend

Do this exercise as described in Series III-3. Repeat 8 times.

IV-4. Arm Circles

Starting position: Stand erect, feet in forward stride position, arms at sides.
Action: Rotate right arm clockwise by moving it in largest circle possible.
Repeat with left arm. Repeat with arms moving alternately. Repeat
15-20 times with each arm.

IV-5. Wing Stretcher 3

Do this exercise as described in Series III-5. Repeat 8-12 times.

IV-6. Body Bender

Do this exercise as described in Series II-5. Do 6 sets.

IV-7. Hamstring Stretch 3

Starting position: Stand erect, feet approximately shoulders' width apart.
Action: While keeping knees straight, stretch body forward with a slow,
sustained stretch and reach between legs, touching the floor behind
your heels. Return to starting position. Repeat 4-8 times, trying to
reach a greater distance behind heels each time.

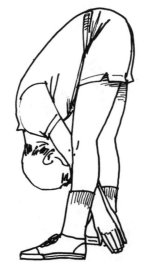

IV-7.   Hamstring Stretch 3

IV-8. Low Back Stretch 1

Do this exercise as described in Series I-8. Repeat 10 times.

IV-9. Low Back Stretch 2

Do this exercise as described in Series III-9. Repeat 8 times.

IV-10. Nose to Knees 1

Do this exercise as described in Series I-9. Repeat 15 times.

IV-11. Nose to Knees 2

Do this exercise as described in Series II-10. Repeat 15 times.

IV-12. Sitting Stride Stretch

Do this exercise as described in Series II-11. Repeat 15-20 times.

IV-13. Tailor Sit 3

Do this exercise as described in Series III-13. Repeat 8-12 times.

IV-14. Hurdle Stretch

Starting position: Sit on floor, left leg extended, right leg bent, knee extended to side with lower leg and foot bent back along buttocks.

Action: Stretch forward, extend hands to left toes, curl head toward knee for a two-second count. Rotate body to right and stretch over bent knee. Return to starting position and repeat 4-8 times. Reverse positions and repeat.

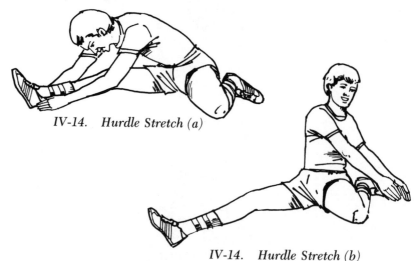

IV-14.   Hurdle Stretch (a)

IV-14.   Hurdle Stretch (b)

IV-15. Heel Cord Stretch 1

Do this exercise as described in Series I-12. Repeat 8 times.

IV-16. Heel Cord Stretch 2

Do this exercise as described in Series III-16. Repeat 8 times.

Strength

IV-17. Head Pull

Do this exercise as described in Series II-15. Repeat 12 times.

IV-18. Pull-ups

Equipment: Securely fastened overhead rope or horizontal bar.
Starting position: Grasp bar with fingers curled toward face.
Action: Pull body up, placing chin over bar. Repeat without touching feet to floor. Do 2-6 pull-ups.

IV-19. Push-ups

Do this exercise as described in Series III-21. Repeat 15-25 times.

IV-20. Chest Raiser 2

Do this exercise as described in Series III-22. Repeat 10-15 times.

IV-21. Abdominal Curls 3

Starting position: Lie on back, knees bent, feet on floor, heels close to buttocks. Clasp hands behind head.
Action: Slowly curl head and shoulders forward for a two-second count. Return to starting position for a two-second count. Repeat 12-30 times.

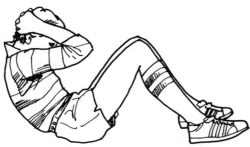

IV-21.   Abdominal Curls 3

IV-22. Leg Raiser 2

Do this exercise as described in Series III-24. Repeat 6-10 times.

IV-23. Side Leg Lift 2

Do this exercise as described in Series III-25. Repeat 10-15 times.

IV-24. Knee Bends

Starting position: Stand erect. arms extended forward shoulder height.
Action: Keep back straight, heels on floor. Bend knees to a 90-degree angle. Return to starting position. Repeat 10-20 times.

IV-25. Wall Sit

Do this exercise as described in Series III-27. Try to increase length of time to two minutes.

IV-26. Ankle Bounce

Starting position: Stand erect, hands on hips.
Action: Bounce in the air with a forceful extension at ankles. Repeat 20-30 times.

SERIES V
Athletic Performance Level

Flexibility

V-1. Head Lift

Starting position: Lie on back on table or bench, head hanging over the edge.
Action: Lift head, bringing chin to chest. Return to starting position. Repeat 8-15 times.

V-2. Arm Circles 2

Starting position: Stand erect, feet in forward stride position, arms at sides.
Action: Swing arms forward and overhead, crossing hands at the wrists, and continuing in large circles sidewards. Make circles as large as possible. Swing with sufficient force to bring feet off floor. Repeat continuously 15-25 times.

V-3. Body Bender

Do this exercise as described in Series II-5, grasping a 3-5 pound weight in each hand. Do 4-6 sets.

V-4. Hamstring Stretch 4

Starting position: Stand erect, feet together, knees straight.

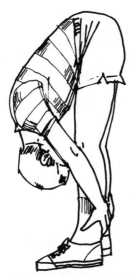

V-4. Hamstring Stretch 4

Action: While maintaining fingers in a locked position, pull head and upper body forward and touch elbows to floor. Return to starting position. Repeat 8-12 times.

V-5. Hamstring Stretch 5

Starting position: Stand erect, feet in wide stride, arms folded across chest.
Action: Bend upper body forward and stretch elbows to the floor. Repeat 4-8 times.

V-6. Seated Leg Lift

Starting position: Sit on floor, leg straight forward, place both hands on one foot.
Action: Bring leg up close to ear. Hold for a four-second count. Return to starting position. Repeat 8-12 times with each leg.

V-7. Sitting Stride Stretch 2

Starting position: Sit on floor, legs in a wide stride position, back erect, fingers interlocked behind head.
Action: While maintaining fingers in a locked position, pull head and upper body forward and touch elbows to floor. Return to starting position. Repeat 8-12 times.

V-8. Sitting Stride Stretch 3

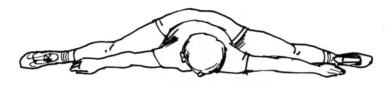

V-8. Sitting Stride Stretch 3

Starting position: Sit on floor, legs in wide stride position, body bent forward with hands on ankles.

Action: Pull body forward, attempting to touch chest to floor. Return to starting position. Repeat up to 25 times.

V-9. Tailor Sit 4

Starting position: Sit on floor, back erect, soles of feet together, in line with knees.

Action: Place hands on knees and gently but firmly press toward floor. Curl head and upper body toward feet. Return to starting position. Repeat 8-12 times.

V-10. Hurdle Stretch

Do this exercise as described in Series IV-14. Repeat 10 times.

V-11. Low Back Stretch 3

Starting position: Lie on back on a table or bench, buttocks close to table edge, one leg hanging over edge. Bend other leg and grasp bent knee with both hands.

Action: Pull knee close to shoulder. Repeat 4-8 times. Change positions and repeat with opposite leg.

V-12. High Kicks

Starting position: Stand erect, arms outstretched shoulder height.

Action: Step forward on right foot and kick left foot up to touch right hand. Repeat by stepping forward on left foot and kicking right foot up to touch right hand. Continue for 20-30 steps.

V-13. Heel Cord Stretch 1

Do this exercise as described in Series I-12. Repeat 8 times with each leg.

V-14. Heel Cord Stretch 2

Do this exercise as described in Series II-14. Repeat 8 times with each leg.

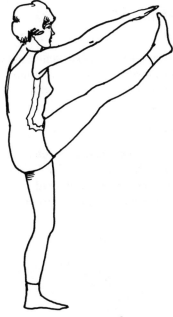

V-12.   High Kicks

Strength

V-15. Head Pull

Do this exercise as described in Series II-15. Repeat 15 times.

V-16. Pull-ups

Do this exercise as described in Series IV-18. Repeat 6-10 times.

V-17. Push-ups

Do this exercise as described in Series III, clapping hands after returning to full extension. Repeat 25-50 times.

V-18. Abdominal Curls 3

Do this exercise as described in Series IV-21. Repeat 30-50 times.

V-19. Abdominal Curls 4

Starting position: Same as 3 with knees shoulder width apart.
Action: Slowly curl head and shoulders diagonally forward bringing left

elbow to outside of right knee. Repeat, bringing right elbow to outside of left knee. Repeat 15-25 times.

V-20. V Curl-ups

Starting position: Lie on back, arms stretched above head.
Action: Curl upper body forward, at the same time bring the feet in the air. Balance on seat while touching toes with hands. Return to starting position. Repeat 10-20 times.

V-21. Back Leg Lift

Starting position: Lie on back, arms outstretched from shoulders.
Action: Raise right leg to the perpendicular. While maintaining arms and shoulders on floor, lower foot to left hand. Return to starting position and repeat by raising left leg and lowering it to right hand. Repeat 10-20 times.

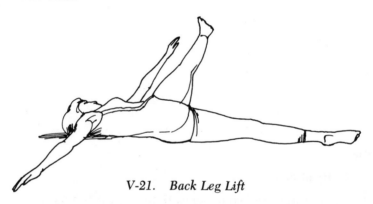

V-21.   Back Leg Lift

V-22. Knee bends

Do this exercise as described in Series IV-24. Repeat 25 or more times.

V-23. Ankle Bounce

Do this exercise as described in Series IV-26. Repeat 20-30 times.

V-24. Tuck Jumping

Starting position: Stand erect.
Action: Jump in the air, bringing knees to a tuck position waist high. Repeat 15-25 times.

Part Two

The Flow and Breath of Life: Cardiovascular Endurance

Jon Livewell has been encouraging his parents to get involved in a cardiovascular endurance exercise program, suggesting that such exercise not only would help them trim off excess pounds but make them feel much better and sleep more soundly. Sharon, the mother, has been bothered lately with insomnia. A family council was held and the entire family decided to plan and engage in cardiovascular endurance exercise programs together. The two chapters in Part Two will describe how the Livewells appraised their cardiovascular endurance levels, and how they planned individualized programs and engaged in those programs. If you follow the same steps the Livewells did, you and your family can have the same success in appraising cardiovascular fitness (Chapter 3) and in planning and engaging in an appropriate cardiovascular endurance program (Chapter 4).

But what is cardiovascular endurance? And why is it so important? *Cardiovascular endurance* is the ability of the heart and lungs to supply needed blood and oxygen to the muscles while they perform work during an extended period of time. Those activities that tend to increase the body's ability to utilize and supply oxygen are called "aerobic" activities. Such activities include walking, jogging, cycling, running in place, swimming, rope jumping, stair climbing, aerobic dance, aerobic ball-handling, basketball, handball, and other activities that require exercise over an extended period of time. As the body is gradually conditioned to engage in such exercises over a long period of time or at a faster rate, physical changes take place in the body that increase your sense of well-being, good health, and efficiency. Some of these changes include:[1]

1. The respiration and heart rate increase less suddenly than was experienced at the beginning of the conditioning program. You don't have to keep stopping to catch your breath. This means the capacity of the lungs is increasing.

2. As you become more conditioned, your heart beats slower but more efficiently, pumping more blood in fewer beats. The average exercise heart beat (the upper limit of an individual's tolerance) is about 150 beats. As fitness improves, the body can tolerate an increased work load without rising above the exercise heart rate.

3. A delay of fatigue and the kind of fatigue that assures sound sleep at night occurs.

4. A more adequate supply of blood to the muscles develops because of a tremendous increase in muscle capillaries. This prevents or considerably reduces muscle soreness, which is the result of an inadequate blood supply to the muscles during exercise.

5. Body muscles are more strengthened and toned because the muscles are larger. (However, women do not become "muscle-bound.") The result is less fatigue for a given amount of activity.

6. Respiratory (breathing) muscles increase in strength and working capacity.

7. The return of blood to the heart from various body parts is greatly facilitated. Veins, which carry blood back to the heart, have valves that prevent the blood from going the wrong direction. The heart's main function is to pump blood away and into the various peripheral regions of the body. Muscles, as they contract, squeeze blood toward the heart. Aerobic exercise increases the size and efficiency of muscles, thus making them

---

[1]Adapted from Harold Shryock M. D., "Is keeping fit a fad?", *Signs of the Times* (October 1969), pp. 26-28.

more effective in their function of squeezing blood toward the heart.

8. Digestion is aided because the increasing flow of blood throughout the digestive organs and glands increases the quantity and flow of digestive juices. Digestion is also aided by the "massaging" action of the muscles — stimulating the flow of food from one organ to another throughout the digestive system.

9. Adequate elimination of waste products from the bowel and the kidneys is promoted. The muscles move the residue toward the large bowel for elimination, and the improved blood circulation provides more efficient function of the kidneys in filtering out waste products from the blood.

10. The onset of some diseases is prevented.

Why all the emphasis on oxygen consumption? What does oxygen consumption have to do with physical fitness? You need oxygen in order to produce energy. If your heart and lungs are working at their most effective and efficient rates, you are capable of utilizing more of the oxygen inhaled with each breath you take, and your heart is capable of pumping more blood with each beat. The result is a lowered breathing and heart rate. Your heart is a magnificent machine. Like any machine, it will last longer if it is kept in good condition and doesn't have to work constantly at top speed. Aerobic exercise allows the heart and lungs to become more effective (do their jobs better) and efficient (do their jobs faster or with less energy expenditure), to work better and longer.

Part Two contains two chapters. Because it is imperative that family members know their individual cardiovascular fitness levels before planning their cardiovascular (aerobics) exercise programs, in Chapter 3 you will learn how to administer and interpret two cardiovascular endurance tests. Once you know the cardiovascular endurance levels of family members, you can plan an individualized cardiovascular endurance exercise program for yourself or any other member of the family. You will learn how to make such programs and engage in them in Chapter 4. The Livewell family will be the focus of the examples used in these two chapters.

Chapter Three

Planning a Cardiovascular Endurance Program

GOAL: Be able to plan a cardiovascular endurance program for yourself or any other member of your family.

Dr. Kenneth Cooper, author of *The New Aerobics*, says the body's ability to take in more oxygen and utilize more oxygen per breath is the best measure of physical fitness. This chapter will help you determine your present fitness level and plan a program that will help you move from your present fitness level to a more desirable one. The emphasis will be on developing your ability to take in more oxygen and utilize more oxygen each time you breath.

The best way to test your fitness level is under some type of stress condition. For instance, how long can you run before you are out of breath? In the exercise laboratory, one such test is walking on a motor-driven treadmill while breathing into a machine that measures exactly how much air you breath in and utilize under stress. Pedaling on a stationary bicycle ergometer is another way to measure your cardiovascular endurance level, but bicycle ergometers are so expensive they are usually found only in health spas or college or university physical education departments.

The tests described in this chapter are not as complicated as those conducted in the laboratory. There is a simple test described later that measures your present heart rate when resting. That resting heart rate is used to determine how to begin your cardiovascular endurance program.

First, a word of caution. You and the other members of your family may be so enthusiastic about getting started on an aerobic exercise program that you may want to skip the cardiovascular tests described in this chapter. Don't! These tests are absolutely essential for each member of the family in determining where to begin an exercise program. It is too easy to get involved in an exercise program that is either too ambitious or not ambitious enough. Either way, your motivation may rapidly diminish because of unexpected pain and oxygen debt (out-of-breath feeling), in the case of an overambitious program, and the feeling of making no progress in the underambitious program. These tests are simple and take relatively little time.

In order for an activity to provide you with cardiovascular benefits, it must be sustained for at least twelve minutes, while keeping your heart rate at or above a certain point. In other words, not all vigorous activity is considered aerobic activity (that is, activity requiring an increased and continuous supply of oxygen over a period of time long enough to produce positive effects on your heart, blood vessels, and lungs — your cardiovascular system). Observe yourself and other members of your family. Are there occasions when you or other family members engage in activities for at least twelve minutes at a time, requiring you to breath hard and your heart to beat much faster than usual? More than likely you won't observe such activity. An occasional quick run up and down the stairs doesn't count. Neither does mowing the lawn, unless you work hard at it for more than twelve minutes at a time. Neither does vacuuming, unless you push for all you're worth for periods of twelve minutes or longer. Neither are a good many sports and recreational activities such as bowling or playing hop scotch or croquet. In order to be physically fit — meaning your cardiovascular endurance level is good to excellent — you must frequently and consistently engage in sustained physical activities that keep your heart rate up for at least twelve minutes at a time.

PROCEDURES

Each member of the family should fill out a separate cardiovascular endurance fitness appraisal form as the procedures in this chapter are followed. As these procedures are described, notice how Jon Livewell's form is filled in (Figure 3-1). Remember that Jon is the sixteen-year-old athlete member of the Livewell family who finally convinced his family to get started on an exercise program.

The first two steps described here are not specific cardiovascular endurance tests. Rather, they are preliminary steps. Step 1 is recommended, step 2 is optional.

STEP 1: *Have a Thorough Medical Examination*

A medical examination for each member of the family is rec-

FIGURE 3-1
CARDIOVASCULAR ENDURANCE
FITNESS APPRAISAL

1. Name __Jon Livewell__ Date _____

Medical Clearance

2. Age ___X___ Under 30: Medical checkup within past year

_____ 30-39: Medical checkup, with resting ECG, within past 3 months

_____ 40-49: Medical checkup, with exercise ECG, within past 3 months

_____ 50+: Same as 40-49, but medical checkup within past week

3. Medical Clearance: No restrictions ___X___ Restrictions (specify) _____

Body Measurements

5. Height __6'4"__
6. Weight __165__
7. Chest __42"__
8. Waist __33"__
9. Hips __40-1/2"__
10. Thigh (right side) __22-1/2"__
11. Calf (right side) __14"__

Resting Heart Rate

9. Day 1 __57__ 10. Day 2 __56__ 11. Day 3 __55__
12. Sum of resting heart rates __168__
13. Add all three heart rates and divide the total by three to determine the resting heart rate __56__

Exercise Heart Rate

14. If a person on line 1 is a child ten years old or younger, write 210; if the person on line 1 is over ten years old, write 220 __220__
15. Write the age of the person on line 1 __16__
16. Maximum Heart Rate (subtract line 15 from line 14) __204__
17. Resting Heart Rate __56__
18. Working Heart Rate (subtract line 17 from line 16) __148__
19. Multiple line 18 by .60; put the answer here __89__
20. Resting Heart Rate (from line 17) __56__
21. Exercise Heart Rate (add line 20 to line 19) __145__

59

ommended before beginning any of the exercise or weight control programs described in this book. Don't let the fact that you and other family members "feel good" prevent any of you from getting an examination. A thorough medical examination can detect the onset of serious illness or disability, the symptoms of which are often mild, undetectable to the person, and present for a long time before they manifest themselves outwardly to indicate something is wrong.

The medical examination should include:

1. chest x-ray
2. blood test (including test for serum cholesterol)
3. urine test
4. blood pressure
5. pap smear test (if adult female)
6. electrocardiogram (ECG) heart tracing (if over age 30): resting ECG if between 30-39, exercise ECG if 40 or older

If any member of the family is under the age of thirty and has had a medical examination within the past year indicating no restrictions, he is ready to move on to step 2. If any member of the family is between the ages of thirty and forty-nine, the medical examination should have occurred within the past two or three months before starting the cardiovascular endurance tests. If any member of the family is over the age of fifty, the medical examination should have occurred within the past week. You should ask the doctor to indicate any limitations or restrictions relative to diet and exercise.

In our illustration, Jon Livewell put his name on line 1 of his cardiovascular endurance fitness appraisal form. Because he is under age thirty and had a medical examination before starting varsity basketball in the fall, he put his age in the "under 30" space in line 2. There were no diet or exercise restrictions made by the doctor at the time of Jon's examination, so Jon checked "no restrictions" on line 3, Medical Clearance.

STEP 2: *Determine Height, Weight, and Girth Measurements*

This step is an optional step. However, people usually discover, as they engage in a cardiovascular endurance (aerobic) exercise program, that several of their body measurements change. The waist and hips slim down and the muscles in the calves and thighs become firmer and perhaps larger, particularly in men. Weight may increase or decrease without a change in eating habits. It is not unusual to gain weight while the waist and hips slim down. This is because muscles are becoming larger and better proportioned. Since muscles weigh more than fat, an increase in weight could be expected. The individual can look better as well as feel better while adding a few more pounds. However, weight loss may also occur. This often depends on the person's body build, eating habits, and amount of exercise. Again, if he feels good and looks good, there is no cause for alarm when weight loss occurs. It is wise to have a record of body measurements before beginning any exercise or diet program in order to check any later changes as the result of diet and exercise. In other words, when you "get there," it's nice to know "where you've been."

The person whose measurements are taken should dress only in underclothes. Someone else should take the measurements.

Height (line 5). The person whose height is being measured should stand straight and flat against a wall that has little floor molding or against a door. Arms should hang loosely at the sides. Mark the wall at the person's tallest point on the head. Use a ruler at a 90-degree angle from the wall, extending it straight across the top of the head to find the tallest point. If the ruler is not at an exact 90-degree angle — that is, parallel to the floor — the measurement will be inaccurate. After the person steps away from the wall or door, use a yardstick or tape measure to measure the distance from the floor to the mark. Write the person's height on line 5 in feet and inches. Jon Livewell's height is six feet two inches (6'2"). Exercise normally does not increase or decrease height, although people have reported increases in height as a result of exercise conditioning.

Weight (line 6). It is best to weigh immediately after rising in the morning because body weight tends to fluctuate throughout the day, depending on how much you eat and what you eat, how active you are, water retention in body tissues, and so on. Use the scale you normally weigh on, such as a bathroom scale. If you use an inexpensive bathroom scale, be sure the pointer is at zero whenever you weigh. Write the number of pounds on line 6. Jon weighs 165 pounds.

Chest (line 7). Make these girth measurements with a standard cloth tape measure, being sure the tape is level around the entire girth area. Stand erect with arms at sides, breathing normally. Place the tape around the chest at nipple level. Write on line 7 the chest measurement in inches. Jon's chest measures forty-two inches.

Waist (line 8). Stand erect, breathing normally, without sucking in or protruding the stomach. Place tape around waist. Write on line 8 the waist measurement in inches. Jon's waist measurement is thirty-three inches.

Hips (line 9). Stand erect with feet together. Place the tape around the largest portion of the hips. Write on line 9 the hip measurement in inches. Jon's hips measure 40½ inches.

Thigh, right side (line 10). Stand erect with feet approximately eighteen inches apart, weight equally distributed. Place the tape around the largest part of the right thigh, which is usually in the crease just below the buttocks. Write on line 10 the right thigh measurement in inches. Jon's right thigh measures 22½ inches.

Calf, right side (line 11). Stand erect with feet approximately eighteen inches apart, weight equally distributed. Place the tape around the largest part of the right calf. Write on line 11 the right calf measurement in inches. Jon's right calf measures fourteen inches.

STEP 3: *Determine Resting Heart Rate*

The heart rate is a basic measure of physical fitness. The faster your heartbeat, the less physically fit you are. A physically fit adult will have a lower heartbeat than the average adult. (This is probably also true for children, but evidence on this is sparse.) However, there is no such thing as an ideal heart rate for everyone. Our normal heart rates are as individual as our fingerprints. The average heart rate for men is less than the average heart rate for women. Women have an average heart rate per minute of about 75, and men have an average heart rate of 70. Children usually have a higher resting heart rate due to rapid growth processes. The normal heart rate also tends to increase with age. So, it is impossible to tell whether your cardiovascular endurance level is excellent, good, fair, or poor simply by finding your average heart rate. The only way you can tell if your cardiovascular endurance level is increasing is to periodically count your resting heart rate during your cardiovascular endurance exercise program. If your resting heart rate is decreasing, you know your cardiovascular endurance level is increasing.

In order to determine your beginning heart rate — from which you will evaluate your fitness level throughout your exercise program — you need to know your resting heart rate before you begin your exercise program.

Before you determine your resting heart rate, it is necessary to practice counting your heart rate. You can count your pulse or heart rate conveniently in two places. One is the cavity of the wrist, about two inches below the base of the thumb radial artery; the other is at the neck on either side of the Adam's apple (carotid artery). Use moderate pressure with the index finger or forefinger to find and count the pulse. Do *not* use the thumb to count pulse rate because it has its own pulse, which may confuse your counting. With a stop watch or a watch or clock with a sweep second hand, practice counting your pulse for fifteen-second and one-minute intervals. Once you think you feel comfortable about finding and counting your pulse rate, do the following to find your resting heart rate:

1.   Count your pulse for exactly one minute immediately following a rest period of at least two hours. The best time to obtain your resting heart rate is just before arising in the morning (be sure you do it *before* you get out of bed and while your heart rate is still low). You will need a stopwatch or a watch or clock with a sweep second hand.

2.   Repeat step 1 three times. The rest periods should be at least twenty-four hours apart. Record each resting heart rate on lines 9, 10, and 11.

3.   Add the three recorded heart rates and record this sum on line 12.

4.   Divide the sum of resting heart rates by 3. This is your average resting heart rate. Record your average resting heart rate on line 13.

Your average resting heart rate will be used throughout your cardiovascular endurance exercise program to evaluate your own individual cardiovascular endurance level improvement.

Unless the child is able to count his or her own heart rate, count the child's heart just as you would your own after each of three two-hour rest periods. Practice counting the child's heart rate before you start the procedures to find the average resting heart rate.

Jon Livewell took his resting heart rate for three days. The first day he had a resting heart rate of 57 (line 9); the second day 56 (line 10); the third day 55 (line 11). The total for the three days was 168 (line 12). He divided line 12 by 3 to determine his resting heart rate, which was 56 (line 13).

STEP 4: *Compute Your Exercise Heart Rate*

We have mentioned the importance of maintaining your heart rate at a certain level in order to achieve cardiovascular benefits from vigorous exercise. This heart rate is unique for every individual, depending on his or her age and resting heart rate. This "magic" heart rate is called your exercise heart rate. Lines 14 through 21 on the cardiovascular endurance fitness appraisal form are designed to help you compute your own exercise heart rate. Here is how you compute it.

Line 14. If you are over ten years of age, write the number 220 on this line. If you are ten years old or younger, write 210 on this line. The explanation for this number is not important for us to understand. It is a number arrived at in laboratory studies in exercise physiology. Jon Livewell is over the age of ten, obviously, so he wrote 220 on line 14 of his appraisal form.

Line 15. Write your age on line 15. If you are preparing this form for someone else, write that person's age on line 15. Jon Livewell wrote his age, sixteen, on line fifteen.

Line 16. In order to find your maximum heart rate (another term used in the laboratory), subtract line 15 from line 14 and write the result on line 16. Jon Livewell subtracted line 15 (16) from line 6 (220) and wrote the result (204) on line 16.

Line 17. Write your resting heart rate from line 13 on line 17.

Line 18. In order to compute your working heart rate (another laboratory term) on line 18, subtract line 17 from line 16. Jon Livewell subtracted line 17 (56) from line 16 (204) and wrote his working heart rate (148) on line 18.

Line 19. Now you are going to use another number derived from laboratory studies. Multiply the number on line 18 by .60. Put the product on line 19. Jon Livewell multiplied line 18 (148) by .60 and the product was 88.8. He rounded this off to the nearest whole number, 89, which he wrote on line 19.

Line 20. This time, write your resting heart rate on line 20. In other words, write on line 20 the same number you wrote on line 13. Jon Livewell wrote 56.

Line 21. Now you are ready to find your own individual exercise heart rate. In order to do this, add line 20 and line 19. Write the sum on line 21. Jon Livewell added line 20 to line 19 and wrote the sum (145) on line 21.

Your exercise heart rate is the rate at which your heart should beat during the sustained exercise of cardiovascular endurance training. When your heart rate during exercise drops below your own special exercise heart rate, it is likely you are not getting any cardiovascular benefit from your exercise unless you increase the length of time you exercise. The whole point of your cardiovascular endurance program is to help you gradually move to the point where you can engage in a desired aerobic activity for at least twelve minutes while your heart pumps away at no less than your own exercise heart rate. But now we move to step 5 to find out where to start on a conditioning program.

STEP 5: *Select a Cardiovascular Endurance Activity*

Cardiovascular endurance (aerobic) activities that all or most members of the family can engage in include: walking, jogging, running in place, stair climbing, rope jumping, swimming, cycling, aerobic ball handling, aerobic dance, and other exercises requiring continuous and vigorous activity. Several of these exercises are described in detail in Chapter 4.

Before you plan *how* you are going to engage in a cardiovascular endurance program, you need to decide *what* cardiovascular endurance activity you want to engage in during your fitness program. If you are unaccustomed to daily sustained vigorous exercise, it may not be wise to engage in more than one type of cardiovascular endurance exercise. Your muscles become accustomed to one type of exercise. You may not be able to maintain your rate of conditioning when you switch from one cardiovascular endurance activity to another. Once you and the other members of the family are in good or excellent condition, you may wish to engage in a variety of cardiovascular endurance activities to add variety and additional pleasure to your program.

Jogging and/or walking[1] is suggested as the best cardiovascular endurance activity to become conditioned. There are several reasons for this. First, jogging can increase your cardiovascular endurance fitness level faster than any other when compared to the amount of time you expend in the activity. For instance, you would have to cycle farther and longer to get the same benefits you would get jogging less distance and time. Many people complain they "don't have time" to engage in vigorous exercise. Compared to other aerobic activities, jogging takes very little time. Second, jogging doesn't require special equipment and facilities. Jogging can be done almost anywhere at any time. The only special requirements are comfortable, durable running shoes with cushion soles and good arch supports and loose-fitting clothing. The family need not spend a great deal of money purchasing special equipment or clothing, nor do they need to spend precious extra minutes traveling to and from a special jogging facility or a track. Third, and possibly most important, all members of the family can participate in jogging. It does not require special skills developed over long hours of practice.

Cardiovascular endurance activities especially well-suited to the participation of all family members together are jogging, rope jumping, aerobic ball handling, and aerobic dance. Other family cardiovascular endurance activities include bicycle riding, swimming, stair climbing, and even racquetball, basketball, and soccer — if the children in the family are old enough to engage in such activities.

---

[1]If you are an older person or find you become overly fatigued with a small amount of running, it may be wise for you to start your fitness program by walking vigorously.

Chapter Four

Engaging in Cardiovascular Endurance Programs

GOAL: Be able to achieve and maintain a cardiovascular endurance level of good or excellent by engaging in your own personalized cardiovascular endurance program.

Chapter 3 has helped you determine the heart rate you should maintain during cardiovascular endurance exercise in order to improve your physical fitness level. In that chapter, you also selected the cardiovascular exercise you wished to engage in. This chapter describes how to begin and how to maintain an effective cardiovascular endurance exercise program.

PROCEDURES

The key phrase for developing physical fitness is "go slow." But "go slow" from where? This section tells you where to begin on a cardiovascular endurance program. You will need to engage in the activity you selected for twelve minutes, so get yourself ready for that activity.

First, warm up and tone up muscles for vigorous activity by engaging in Series I strength and flexibility exercises. Second, practice counting your heart rate. You need to have a stopwatch or clock with a second hand. To determine the speed at which you should exercise, start with a brisk walk. After walking about one minute, *stop*, and while standing, count your pulse for exactly fifteen seconds. Multiply that number by four to determine the exercise heart rate per minute (4 x 15 seconds = 60 seconds = 1 minute). Compare this number with your computed exercise heart rate (line 21 on the cardiovascular endurance fitness appraisal you completed in Chapter 3). If your present heart rate is *higher* than the number from line 21, you should slow down but continue walking. If your present heart rate is lower than the number from line 21, you should speed up your pace. Continue walking and monitoring your heart every one to two minutes until you have found the speed at which you should walk in order to maintain your own exercise heart rate (line 21).

Once you have achieve your computed exercise heart rate, note your breathing and how you feel. Use this as an indicator for maintaining the same level of activity for each two-minute period of vigorous activity. When you become fatigued, walk until the heart rate slows down to 120. Then repeat the exercise. Continue the run-walk pattern for a total of twelve minutes of activity at your computed exercise heart rate. When exercising with friends or family members, maintain your own pace rather than attempting to compete with or match their pace.

Avoid pushing yourself to a point of overfatigue. Some signs of overwork are chest pain, dizziness or light headedness, severe breathlessness, nausea, or extreme weakness of muscles. Your heart rate should fall below 120 beats per minute within five minutes after exercise and below 100 within ten minutes after exercise. Progress slowly so that your body can adjust to its new exercise program.

You will note that your heart rate will slow down to 120 in a shorter period of time as your cardiovascular condition improves, and that you can maintain the exercise heart rate for a longer period of time. Your goal is to be able to run for twelve minutes covering a distance of 1 to 1½ miles. During the cardiovascular exercise, the heel cord stretching exercise (wall push-away) described in Series I strength and flexibility exercises should be used in the event pain is felt between the calf of the leg and the heel.

The walk-jog program just described, where you walk for a while when you become fatigued, while jogging at your computed exercise heart rate, is designed to help your body adjust to vigorous exercise. If you start on a cardiovascular endurance program by attempting to maintain your exercise heart rate for a full twelve minutes, you will likely find that you experience great pain and fatigue — and discouragement. The body needs time to adjust to a new exercise program. Do the walk-jog program until you can maintain a jog for twelve minutes at your exercise heart rate without becoming unduly fatigued. Gradually increase the amount of time you jog and decrease the amount of time you walk until you have eliminated walking.

The purpose of maintaining your exercise heart rate during a twelve-minute period is to allow conditioning effects to take place in the body as a result of the exercise. If you fall below your computed exercise heart rate during each twelve-minute period of activity, it is not likely your body will gain full benefit from the exercises. That is, you may expend a few calories, but your heart and lungs will not become more efficient in their use of oxygen.

Once you have reached the point where you can engage in your desired cardiovascular endurance activity (CVE) for twelve minutes at your exercise heart rate, you may then concentrate on increasing your exercise heart rate. Figures 4-1 to 4-3 show the heart rate conditioning zone for persons of any sex at any given age. Your heart rate conditioning zone is the interval between your first computed exercise heart rate (the one you computed for line 21 on your CVE appraisal in Chapter 3) and the suggested maximum exercise heart rate if you are in excellent physical condition. For instance, Jon Livewell is sixteen (closer to fifteen on the chart in Figure 4-1). His heart rate conditioning zone would be an exercise heart rate between 152 and 185.[1] This means his exercise heart rate should not go below 152 during exercise and, once he is in good physical condition, can increase to as high as 185. If he engages in vigorous exercise for twelve minutes at a higher exercise heart rate than 185, he may experience extreme fatigue, which can be harmful to the body. Well-conditioned athletes, however, exercise frequently at the higher levels when they are in preparation for competition.

As you become more physically fit, you will find that it takes longer for your exercise heart rate to occur. That means your heart is pumping more blood with each beat, and the lungs are utilizing more oxygen from any given amount of blood so it takes more vigorous exercise to get the heart rate up to its minimum conditioning level. This means, as you become more physically fit, you must engage in your cardiovascular endurance activity for a longer period of time.

When you finish your exercise period each day, be sure to cool down by engaging in the exercise slowly for four to five minutes. If you follow this routine, you will enjoy a more pleasant and pain-free cardiovascular endurance program. Specific procedures for a variety of endurance exercises are described in the pages that follow.

JOGGING

Here are a few points to make jogging a pleasant as well as a healthful experience:

---

[1]Jon Livewell's resting heart rate on his CVE appraisal form is 56, considerably lower than the national average of 70 for males. Thus his exercise heart rate on that form actually starts at 145 instead of 152, indicated in Figure 4-1.

FIGURE 4-1
GENERAL CONDITIONING ZONE

Male
(Computed at the average resting
heart rate of 70)

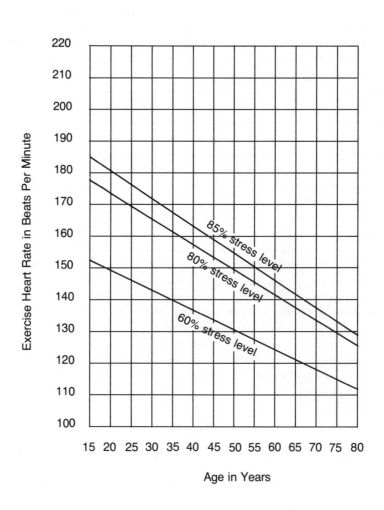

FIGURE 4-2
GENERAL CONDITIONING ZONE

Female
(Computed at the average resting
heart rate of 75)

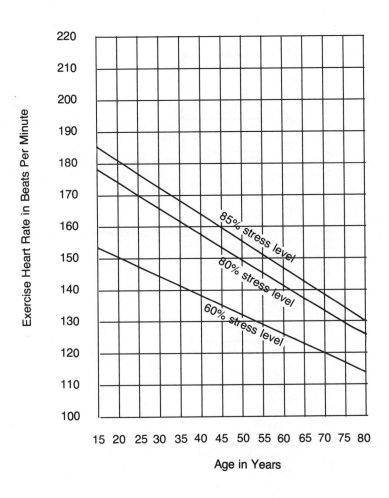

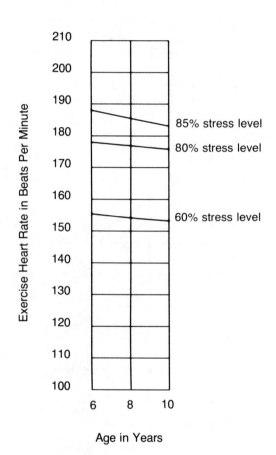

FIGURE 4-3
GENERAL CONDITIONING ZONE

Children to Ten Years of Age
(Computed at the average resting
heart rate of 80)

Age in Years

1. The stride should be loose and natural with no tension in the arms or torso.
2. Look straight ahead while jogging, not at your feet.
3. Maintain an upright position while jogging, leaning neither forward nor back.
4. Bend the arms at the elbow and move them rhythmically in an easy swing back and forth at the sides, not in front, of the body.
5. Move the legs in an easy rhythmic movement from the hips.
6. Breathe naturally with the mouth open.
7. The shoe can hit the ground in either of two ways, whichever is most comfortable: heel to toe — land on the heel of the foot and rock the body forward to the toe; flat foot — strike the entire bottom of the foot against the jogging surface at the same instant. The foot just barely clears the ground as it is lifted for each stride.

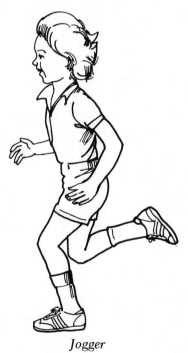

Jogger

What to Wear

Clothing should always be loose-fitting to allow for the full range of body movement. On warm days wear light, heat-reflecting clothing. On cold days wear warm, heat-preserving clothing. Regardless of the temperature, clothing should allow for evaporation of perspiration. Therefore, avoid plastic or rubberized clothes.

Socks should fit well, be soft and absorbent, and thick for protection and comfort. Shoes are the most important item for jogging. Don't spare expense on jogging shoes. The soles should be pliable and cushioned (such as sponge or ripple sole), yet firm, and provide good friction on the jogging surface to prevent slipping or sliding. The shoes should fit well (try them on with the socks you plan to wear with them). They should have a solid heel and a good arch support.

Where to Jog

It is possible for almost anyone to find a good place to jog. A fancy track or grass or jogging path is not necessary, although such places may be more motivating for some people. For the beginning jogger, a softer surface, such as turf, is preferable to cement, particularly for those who are susceptible to pains and aches. However, even cement hazards can be minimized if you wear proper shoes, condition yourself gradually, and carefully follow your own individualized cardiovascular endurance program.

It is easier to measure distance on a track than on streets, paths, park lawns, etc. However, you can pick a favorite place to jog and measure it by the amount of time it takes you to cover a given distance, such as a mile. If the weather is bad, you can jog around a room or in the basement (or even around the inside of the garage if it isn't a cluttered obstacle course). You can use a treadmill or stationary bicycle in the family room or recreation room while you listen to your favorite music or watch television. You can jog in place if the weather is bad, as long as you stay within your heart rate conditioning zone for twelve minutes or longer. Jogging in place has the disadvantage of not using hip muscles as fully as jogging outdoors.

When to Jog

Any time of the day is acceptable, with two exceptions. First, do not jog for at least 1½ hours after a meal. Second, do not jog in the middle of a hot, humid day.

Some families jog before breakfast to get them started on a good day. Other families prefer the noon hour when they can exercise and eat a light meal. Other families prefer to jog before dinner to overcome the tensions and fatigue of the day and receive that extra psychological and physical boost important for the activities of the evening. Some families prefer to jog just before bedtime to relax and sleep better. However, it is not a good idea to jog in unlighted areas because of hazards, such as stepping on small stones, that could result in a sprained ankle or a broken leg. And, it is better to jog at the same time each day. You must plan it in your schedule, or your jogging time will get taken up with other activities. Jog at least four times a week, allowing no more than forty-eight hours to slip by between exercise periods.

Jogging Speed

After you have engaged in a gradual conditioning program, you should jog fast enough to achieve and maintain your own individualized exercise heart rate (see Chapter 3) for twelve minutes per exercise period.

Competition and Jogging

Jogging is not a competitive activity except against your own previous performance. If family members start competing with each other, jogging soon becomes running, and even sprinting, both of which are useless for family members, because the desired length of the activity period usually cannot be maintained, and because it can result in painful shin-splints, sore ankles, swollen knees, and even heart attacks for adults who are not yet physically fit. Because members of any family vary considerably in age, competition among family members is usually unfair because of differences in maturation, muscular and skeletal structure, length of stride, heart rate, and interest in the activity. If a family member is competing with his own previous record, he should immediately slow down or even stop if he becomes aware of any feeling of undue breathlessness, faintness, or pain.

Age and Jogging

If there is no medical indication otherwise, jogging is appropriate for all ages. That means a child can start jogging as soon as he is able to run without losing his balance. If a family member is over fifty and has been living a sedentary life for several years, he should confine exercise to walking for at least three months when beginning an exercise program. Some people should never go beyond walking. If a person over fifty learns to walk briskly without undue breathlessness or feeling of body distress and pain, the advance to slow jog is usually quite simple and easy. Family members who have gradually conditioned themselves to frequent strenuous exercise can maintain their capability by engaging in that exercise at least four times a week.

Sex Differences and Jogging

Heart rate, length of stride, and center of gravity are the major differences between the sexes in any cardiovascular endurance exercise. The heart rate of the average woman and girl is usually higher than that of the man or boy of the same age. This means a well-conditioned mother will have a lower heart rate than when she started vigorous exercise, but her heart rate will still be higher than that for her well-conditioned husband. Because heart rate tends to increase with age, it is a useless exercise to compare the heart rates among children in the family, except to note that they may be the same as each other or different from one another.

Because males tend to have a longer stride than females of the same age, a man and woman can run at the same pace but the man will be ahead of the woman. Because a woman's center of gravity is lower than that of the average man, she may need to expend more energy per jogging stride to propel herself forward.

Pain When Jogging

If you are just starting your jogging program, it is normal to feel some aches and pains in tendons, joints, and ligaments, because unused muscles are now being exposed to vigorous activity. Remember that your legs bear most of the strain and tension during movement. If your muscles are strained or injured, rather than just sore and stiff, you are probably jogging too fast and/or too long, or perhaps you are not jogging in correct body form.

Occasionally a person will get sore heels when jogging. This can be due either to the shoes or to the way the person is jogging. Shoes should cushion the stress on the heels and ankles when running. If you are running by hitting the ground heel first, try the flat-footed approach, which is usually more successful. Shoes should have thick but resilient soles. Ripple soles are great. If you like or need arch supports in jogging shoes, use them. Most pain can be avoided if you remember to warm up with flexibility and strength exercises before jogging, to cool down afterward, and to wear proper shoes. If you experience pain in your legs during jogging, stop and do the heel cord stretch exercise.

Jogging on Streets and Roadways

Heed the following precautions if you and the family jog on streets and roadways: (a) avoid rush hours; (b) always face oncoming traffic; (c) if jogging as a group, jog in single file; (d) wear bright colors during the day, white at night; (e) run only when there is enough light to see clearly; (f) run in place at home when the weather is bad (or jog around the room or use the stationary bicycle, etc.).

JUMPING ROPE

Obtain a rope suitable for jumping, such as a ⅜-inch cord. A commercially made rope with handles can be purchased at a sporting goods or department store. To determine the length, stand on the center of the rope and bring the ends to your armpits on each side.

Remember to warm up before beginning your rope jumping. It is especially important to condition your legs and feet beforehand. Exercises for strengthening the feet and the heel cord stretch should be performed prior to and during the rope jumping activity.

When jumping rope, land lightly on the balls of your feet. The feet should not make any noise as they contact the floor. This will prevent jarring and consequent tearing of the muscle fibers and possible shin splints. Land on both feet at the same time, or on one foot alternating left and right. Jump 50-60 jumps per minute and then walk for one minute. Repeat two or three times. Try to attain 2½ minutes during each day during the first week. Increase your rope jumping time by 2½ minutes during each subsequent two-week period and gradually decrease the walking time until you are jumping continuously. That is, by the end of the third week you should be jumping 5 minutes daily; by the end of the fifth week you should be jumping 7½ minutes daily. Continue this gradual increase until you are jumping 12 to 15 minutes daily. Monitor your heart rate as described in Chapter 3.

Learning a variety of jump rope skills will allow you to move about and to vary the speed of performance and the amount of stress placed on any body part. It is important that you perform skills that you have mastered, skills that can be performed at various tempos, and skills that will not place undue stress on any part of the body. Combine these skills in a sequence that will produce the desired exercise heart rate. Repeat the sequence for a minimum of twelve minutes in order to achieve a cardiovascular training effect (once you have become conditioned to jumping that long). You may wish to select music for accompaniment to increase your enjoyment of your rope jumping activity. You can select jump rope skills from among the following, which are presented in order of difficulty. However, a given skill may be more difficult for one person than for another. Each person should select the skills that seem easiest to perform and then move to those that are more challenging.

A. Beginning Skills

1. Double Bounce — Feet rebound from the floor twice with each revolution of the rope.
2. Single Bounce — Feet rebound from the floor once with each revolution of the rope.
3. Alternate Double Bounce and Single Bounce — Feet rebound once with a revolution of the rope followed by a double bounce on the next revolution.
4. Double Bounce on Alternate Foot — Rebound twice on right foot followed by a double rebound on left foot.
5. Alternate Double and Single Bounce — A double bounce on right foot and single bounce on left foot.
6. Forward Kick — Using a double rebound, kick forward, alternating right and left foot.
7. Stride Jump — Rebound over the rope and land with feet about twelve to fifteen inches apart. On the next revolution land with feet together.
8. Stride Cross — Rebound over the rope and land with feet about twelve inches apart. On the next revolution land with right foot crossed in front of left foot.
9. Criss-Cross — Rebound over the rope and land with right foot crossed in front of the left foot. On the next revolution land with left foot crossed in front of right foot.
10. Indian Stomp — While performing a double rebound on right foot, touch ball of left foot to the floor and raise it quickly by bringing the knee high in the air. Repeat several times on right foot followed by several repetitions on left foot.
11. Heel Touch — Rebound over the rope and land with weight on left foot. At the same time touch right heel forward. On the next revolution land with weight on right foot and touch left heel forward.
12. Toe Touch — Rebound over the rope and land with weight on left foot. At the same time lightly tap toe of right foot behind left heel. On the next revolution land with weight on right foot and tap left toe behind right heel.
13. Heel-Toe Touch Variations —
    a. On the first revolution touch right heel in front. On the next revolution touch left toe behind. Repeat in like manner for several revolutions.
    b. On the first revolution touch right heel. On the next revolution touch right toe. Repeat alternating right foot and left foot.
    c. With one revolution of the rope touch right heel followed im-

mediately by touching right toe. On the second revolution repeat by touching left heel and toe.

d.   On each revolution tap toe twice alternating right and then left.

B. Traveling Skills

1.   Combination
   a.   Perform the double bounce on both feet traveling forward with each revolution of the rope.
   b.   Perform the double bounce alternating right and left foot by taking a step forward with each revolution of the rope.
   c.   Run forward by performing a single rebound on alternate feet.
   d.   Run forward taking two steps on each revolution of the rope.
2.   Hop — Rebound over the rope on each revolution several times on right foot. Repeat with left foot.
3.   Skip over the Rope — The skip is accomplished by hopping over the rope with right foot followed by a hop over the rope on the next revolution with left foot. Repeat.
4.   Twosies — Hop over the rope on the first two revolutions with right foot. On the next two revolutions hop over the rope with left foot. The rope should be turned rapidly to perform a single rebound with each revolution.
5.   Gallop — Complete a gallop with each revolution of the rope. Lead with right foot stepping over the rope and left foot being brought up to right foot. The lead foot remains the same for several repetitions. Change lead foot by making a hop.
6.   Slide — Both feet go over the rope as they are brought together on the slide. Step sideward right with right foot bringing left foot to right foot. Continue in the same direction for several repetitions.
7.   Leap — Leap over the rope by projecting the body in the air. By necessity, the turn of the rope will be slowed down from that of the run.

C. Intermediate Skills

1.   Backward Turning Rope — Perform each of the skills listed under Beginning Skills while turning the rope over the head from front to back.
2.   Traveling Skills
   a.   Perform Traveling Skills with a backward turning rope. Continue to travel in a forward direction.
   b.   Perform Traveling Skills with a backward turning rope, traveling in a backward direction.

3. Cross Arms
    a. Perform either a double or single bounce as you turn the rope by crossing arms in front of the body on the first revolution of the rope and uncrossing on the second revolution. Repeat.
    b. Repeat Cross Arms with a backward turning rope.

D. Dance Skills

1. Two-Step — Step over the rope with right foot on the first revolution and do a ball change, freeing left foot to step over the rope on the next revolution and repeat the ball change. (Ball change: take weight on the ball of the foot momentarily and then shift weight to the opposite foot.)
2. Samba — Step forward over the rope on the first revolution and perform a ball change. Step backward over the rope on the next revolution and perform a ball change. Continue in the same manner, moving shoulders and head back as the forward step is taken and moving shoulders and head forward as the backward step in taken.
3. Pony — Leap over the rope with right foot on the first revolution and perform a ball change. Bring the knees high on each move to maintain the "pony" style. Repeat by leaping over the rope with left foot on the next revolution.
4. Grapevine
    a. Step over the rope on the first revolution by crossing right foot in front of left. Step left on left foot. On the next revolution cross right foot behind left foot and step left with left foot. Repeat, moving to the side in the same direction.
    b. Perform as directed above with the rope turning twice as fast so a revolution is completed on each step.
5. Polka — Hop over the rope on the first revolution with right foot and perform a step-together-step. Hop over the rope on the second revolution with left foot and perform a step-together-step. The rope will need to be turned slowly in order to perform the four-count polka with each revolution.
6. Pas de Basque — Leap to the right with right foot on the first revolution. Bring left foot in front of right foot to perform a ball change. Repeat by leaping to the left with left foot and bringing right foot in front of left foot to perform a ball change.
7. Flea Hop
    a. With weight on right foot lift left foot and hop sideward left. With weight on left foot lift right foot and hop sideward right. Repeat. Complete one revolution of the rope with each hop.

  b. Doubles — With weight on right foot lift left foot and hop sideward left. Tap left foot to floor, at the same time hop sideward to left again. Repeat by alternating to left and right. Complete one revolution of the rope with each hop.

8. Tap Dance
  a. Step Brush — Step over the rope with left foot on the first revolution, brush ball of right foot to floor with a forward motion. Repeat by stepping over the rope with right foot and brushing left foot forward.
  b. Singles — Move forward over the rope alternating right and left with a slap step.
  c. Doubles — Step over the rope with left foot and slap ball of right foot forward and back. Repeat by stepping over rope with right foot and slapping ball of left foot forward and back.
  d. Double Ball Change — Step over the rope with left foot, slap forward and back with right foot, perform a ball change. Repeat by stepping over the rope on the second revolution with right foot and perform a ball change. The rope will need to be turned slowly in order to complete one double ball change on each revolution.

E. Advanced Skills

1. Cut Step — Rebound over the rope with left foot at the same time swinging right leg sideward right. Repeat by rebounding over the rope on right foot while lifting left foot sideward left.
2. Double Unders — Turn the rope twice while making one rebound.
3. Triple Unders — Turn the rope three times while making one rebound.
4. Bells — On the first revolution, rebound over the rope by crossing right leg in front of left. On the second revolution, raise left leg sideward to left and bring right leg sideward to left, clicking heels together. Repeat by crossing left leg in front of right on the next revolution of the rope. On the following revolution, raise right leg sideward to right and bring left leg sideward to right, clicking heels together.

AEROBIC BALL HANDLING

An interesting variation of cardiovascular endurance activity is bouncing a ball, especially if members of the family are basketball fans or participants in that sport. Dribbling a ball while performing such locomotor skills as running, sliding, jumping, hopping, leaping, galloping, and skipping can increase ball handling skills as well as cardiovascular endurance. The person can also dribble with the right hand, dribble with the left hand, and dribble with alternate right and left hands. Use various combinations of the following locomotor skills for dribbling sequences:

1. Walk forward
2. Walk backward
3. Run forward
4. Run backward
5. Slide to the right
6. Slide to the left
7. Skip forward
8. Skip backward
9. Run in different patterns: circles, zig-zag, etc.
10. Run at varying tempos
11. Jump while shooting the ball in the air and catch it before it hits the floor

As with any other cardiovascular endurance activity, monitor your heart rate to make certain you maintain your exercise heart rate for at least twelve minutes (after you become conditioned to this period of time). Repeat the activity at least four times a week. Allow no more than forty-eight hours between ball-handling activity periods.

AEROBIC DANCE

Aerobic dance refers to vigorous movements performed to music. The movements, or dance steps, which can be quite simple, are arranged (choreographed) into interesting sequences requiring a high energy level to produce a cardiovascular training effect.

How to Get Started

Select any one or combination of locomotor movements such as walking, running, leaping, hopping, jumping, galloping, sliding, and skipping. You can add variety and interest by applying some of the elements of space, such as changing direction, increasing the range of movement, changing body levels, varying formation to give interesting floor patterns or designs, and so forth. You can also add strength and flexibility exercises of a vigorous nature such at straddle-hops, toe touches, side benders, and so on (see Chapter 2).

How to Arrange Sequences (Choreograph)

The following simple procedures will help you arrange sequences for aerobic dance activities:

1. Keep the steps simple. Remember, the purpose is to develop

cardiovascular endurance. If the steps are difficult, the performer will be slowed down.

2. Plan to repeat each step four, eight, sixteen, or thirty-two times in order to simplify the activity.
3. Place the steps in logical sequence and repeat the sequences.
4. Select a popular tune with good 2/4, 3/4, or 4/4 rhythm, one that has a catchy beat. Then perform the aerobic dance routine to the music. Here is an example of one such routine to 4/4 music:

FIGURE 4-4
DANCE SEQUENCE

Sequence	Count	Steps
I	16	Jog forward in circle (counterclockwise)
	16	Jog backward (clockwise)
	8	Straddle hops (make 1/2 turn while jumping) facing center
	8	Straddle hops facing out
II	16	Slide right
	8	Alternate heel touch in front
	16	Slide left
	8	Alternate heel touch in front
III	8	Toe Touch (right hand to left toe; repeat left hand to right toe)
	8	Push-ups
	16	Jump in place (4 jumps facing each direction)
IV		Repeat from beginning

The dance sequence can be much simpler than this, such as only four or five steps in a sequence repeated over and over. You can choreograph your own routines to add variety and interest. During the dance activity remember to monitor your heart and maintain your exercise heart rate for at least twelve minutes (once you are conditioned to dance that long).

If your family likes to engage in cardiovascular endurance activities together, be sure to plan activities that all members can participate in. The timing of your exercise is important. You should exercise at least four times a week and space your sessions so they are not more than forty-eight hours apart. Avoid exercising immediately (one-two hours) after eating.

About once a month or every six weeks after you begin your cardiovascular conditioning program, fill out another cardiovascular endurance fitness appraisal form by taking body measurements and determining your resting heart rate and your exercise heart rate. Compare the new computations with the previous form you completed. You may notice that some body measurements have increased, some have decreased, or your resting heart rate may be lower. If so, this will change your exercise heart rate.

A month or six weeks into your cardiovascular endurance program, you will also be ready to take the twelve-minute jog-walk test to measure your cardiovascular endurance level. This is an adaptation of a simple test developed by Dr. Kenneth Cooper in his book, *The New Aerobics.* Use a stopwatch or a regular watch with a sweep second hand. Wear comfortable running shoes and loose-fitting clothing. This test is best done with a partner who does the timing and measuring.

1. Determine the length of the area where you will take the test. Most school tracks are one-quarter mile in length. Or, you can mark off every eighth of a mile (fifty-five yards) in any other area of your choice.

2. Warm up just before testing for five-seven minutes using gradual stretching exercises (no bouncing please, or you'll be sore for sure).

3. To begin the test, run at a slow to moderate pace. When you feel out of breath, stop running and walk until your breathing comes easier. Then continue running again. Keep doing this run-walk procedure for exactly twelve minutes.

4. Figure out the distance you covered in twelve minutes by adding together the number of laps or smaller segments.

5. Using the amount of distance covered, find your cardiovascular fitness category (rating) by referring to the appropriate chart in Figure 4-5.

Cautions:

1. *Stop* running or walking if you experience any pain or dizziness. Do not continue the test.

2. An all-out effort to cover the distance in as short a time as possible is dangerous and, therefore, not advisable. Such sudden exertion can result at worst in a heart attack and at best in sore muscles and respiratory problems. You probably will not be able to finish the test if you give it an all-out effort. You are

FIGURE 4-5
TWELVE-MINUTE WALKING/RUNNING TEST
Distance (Miles) Covered in 12 Minutes

Fitness Category			Age (Years)				
		13-19	20-29	30-39	40-49	50-59	60+
I. Very poor	(men)	<1.30*	<1.22	<1.18	<1.14	<1.03	<.87
	(women)	<1.0	<.96	<.94	<.88	<.84	<.78
II. Poor	(men)	1.30-1.37	1.22-1.31	1.18-1.30	1.14-1.24	1.03-1.16	.87-1.02
	(women)	1.00-1.18	.96-1.11	.95-1.05	.88-.98	.84-.93	.78-.86
III. Fair	(men)	1.38-1.56	1.32-1.49	1.31-1.45	1.25-1.39	1.17-1.30	1.03-1.20
	(women)	1.19-1.29	1.12-1.22	1.06-1.18	.99-1.11	.94-1.05	.87-.98
IV. Good	(men)	1.57-1.72	1.50-1.64	1.46-1.56	1.40-1.53	1.31-1.44	1.21-1.32
	(women)	1.30-1.43	1.23-1.34	1.19-1.29	1.12-1.24	1.06-1.18	.99-1.09
V. Excellent	(men)	1.73-1.86	1.65-1.76	1.57-1.69	1.54-1.65	1.45-1.58	1.33-1.55
	(women)	1.44-1.51	1.35-1.45	1.30-1.39	1.25-1.34	1.19-1.30	1.10-1.18
VI. Superior	(men)	>1.87	>1.77	>1.70	>1.66	>1.59	>1.56
	(women)	>1.52	>1.46	>1.40	>1.35	>1.31	>1.19

* < Means "less than"; > means "more than."

From *The Aerobics Way* by Kenneth H. Cooper, M.D., M.P.H. Copyright © 1977 by Kenneth H. Cooper. Reprinted by permission of the publisher, M. Evans and Company, Inc., New York, N.Y. 10017.

simply trying to find out your cardiovascular endurance level — not trying to beat the world's record in long-distance running.

This run-walk test measures your work capacity. In other words, it is a measure of the amount of blood your heart can pump with each beat and the capacity of your lungs to utilize the oxygen you take in. The higher your cardiovascular endurance level, the more blood your heart is capable of pumping with each beat, and the more oxygen your lungs are capable of using with each breath. That is, the higher your cardiovascular endurance level, the longer you can endure strenuous physical activity.

After you begin your cardiovascular conditioning program, regardless of the exercise you choose, periodically test yourself with this same twelve-minute jog-walk test to check your progress. Your goal should be at least the good category.

FREQUENTLY ASKED QUESTIONS

1. *If a member of our family is overweight, can he or she merely engage in a cardiovascular endurance program in order to lose weight, or is a diet essential?*

Overweight is the result of taking in more calories than are burned up. Cardiovascular endurance exercises burn calories. If you eat no more calories per day after you start your cardiovascular endurance program than you did before you were exercising, you will probably lose weight. However, if a person wishes to lose weight, exercise plus diet is recommended (see Chapter 6 for diet recommendations) because a greater loss of body fat will occur. Dieting alone is likely to result in a loss of muscle tissue with fat. Loss of fat is the purpose of dieting, not loss of muscle tissue.

2. *What effect will cardiovascular endurance activity have on my appetite?*

Contrary to what most people think, vigorous exercise generally does not result in increased appetite. As a matter of fact, most people have very little appetite immediately following a vigorous exercise period. Of course, if the person engages in a great deal of exercise, such as an athlete, there will be increased food intake to maintain the nutrition for strength of the body.

3. *I gained five pounds after I started my cardiovascular endurance program. However, I've never felt so good. Should I try to lose those five pounds I gained?*

You might have gained muscle tissue but lost body fat. Muscle tissue is more dense than body fat, so your body dimensions may have become smaller because of the loss of fat, in spite of your gain in weight. To find out whether or not you need to try to lose those five pounds, check your percent body fat as explained in Chapter 5.

4. *Can I develop cardiovascular endurance by doing calisthenics?*

With the possible exception of stationary running and jumping up and down, most calisthenics exercises are engaged in for far too short a time period to provide cardiovascular benefits. Not only must the activity be engaged in for at least twelve minutes, but you must maintain your exercise heart rate throughout that period. Calisthenics do develop cardiovascular endurance if planned carefully to maintain your exercise heart rate for at least twelve minutes each exercise period.

5. *If I achieve good cardiovascular endurance, will I avoid a heart attack?*

There is no way to guarantee immunity from a heart attack. However, inactivity is a high risk factor related to heart disease. Cardiovascular fitness will decrease your chances of having a heart attack, will decrease the severity of a heart attack if you have one, and will increase your chances of survival.

6. *What do I do if I get a pain in my side while I'm exercising?*

Slow down your exercise pace until the pain decreases. *Don't* stop unless the pain is so severe you can't keep going. Although the exact cause of such pain is not known, one theory is that it is caused by trapped metabolic gases creating increased pressure and, thus, pain. (This can often be relieved by exhaling forcefully.) Another theory is that the respiratory muscles are not getting enough oxygen. As you continue with your cardiovascular endurance program and your fitness level improves, this problem in most cases will be eliminated.

7. *What are shin splints?*

When the muscles and/or tendons of the lower leg become inflamed, this is called shin splints. They are usually caused by running on surfaces that are too hard, running in shoes that do not have proper arch supports, or by engaging in strenuous activity without prior conditioning. Good stretching warm-up exercises before cardiovascular endurance activity may eliminate this problem. If stretching exercises do not help, discontinue your program until the legs heal.

8. *Which is better, to run on a soft surface or a hard surface? Is jogging on the beach in the sand good cardiovascular endurance activity?*

Generally it is better to run on a soft surface than a hard surface — to reduce the stress on joints and connective tissue. Your shoes are all-important when jogging. If you have a good pair of shoes, they will absorb the shock of your running regardless of the hardness of the surface. Running in the sand on the beach is an enjoyable activity, but you may find that you need to increase your running time because of the resistance of the sand.

9. *Why do I perspire more after I jog than while I'm jogging?*

During the vigorous exercise, the focus of your blood flow is to the muscle tissues of the skeleton. This means blood is shunted away from the skin. But when you run, a great deal of heat is generated when the blood focuses on the muscles instead of the skin. When you slow down and finally stop, the blood flows with greater profusion to your skin, causing you to perspire as the body gives off its excess heat. You perspire during jogging, but your perspiration evaporates to a great extent during such vigorous activity.

10. *How am I supposed to breathe when I jog?*

Breathe the way you always breathe, naturally and normally. Holding your breath or trying to regulate your breathing does not contribute to easier breathing or to cardiovascular fitness. Incidentally, huffing and puffing during exercise is normal, not a sign of lack of fitness.

11. *What do we do about our cardiovascular endurance program if the family takes a vacation or someone becomes ill?*

It is generally not wise to exercise if you are ill. Cardiovascular benefits gained in a conditioning program can be lost in two weeks if stopped altogether. This is why it is recommended that you exercise at least four times a week to maintain your fitness level. Even though a vacation means a change from your normal routine, in most cases it is still possible to engage in vigorous activity such as stair climbing, running in place, or rope jumping.

12. *I have heard that a cool down is necessary after vigorous activity. Why is this important and how do you cool down?*

The cool down is absolutely essential after vigorous aerobic activity. The large muscles of the body provide a pumping action that helps circulate the blood back to the heart. Because of the extra load on the heart, without this pumping action of the muscles the venous blood may pool or stagnate and not get back to the heart. Continuing the activity at a slower pace, gradually coming to a slow walk, will allow the body to return to a normal function while the muscles move, thus exerting the necessary pumping action.

CARDIOVASCULAR ENDURANCE ACTIVITY LOG

Members of the family may wish to keep individual cardiovascular endurance activity logs similar to the one in Figure 4-6. After filling in your name, date, age, beginning resting heart rate (from your cardiovascular endurance fitness appraisal which you completed in Chapter 3), and the activity or activities you have selected for your cardiovascular endurance program, you can fill in the remainder of the log as you exercise each

FIGURE 4-6

CARDIOVASCULAR ENDURANCE ACTIVITY LOG

Name —————————————————— Date ————————— Age ————

Beginning Resting Heart Rate ——————————————

Activities: ——————————————

Week	Date	Day	Activity	Duration/Distance, etc.

day. Column 1 refers to each week of the program. Column 2 refers to each day of the month you exercise. The third column is the day of the week on which you complete the exercise (Monday, Wednesday, etc.). Column 4 is the name of the activity (that is, jogging, rope jumping, etc.). The fifth column refers to the distance and/or duration in which you engaged in the activity that day.

You should follow a consistent cardiovascular endurance program. Your log helps you to keep track of your progress, to determine whether or not you are adhering to your cardiovascular endurance program at any given period of time, and can be a reinforcer to continue your program, especially if the log is displayed where others can see it. A word of caution. Do not use your log to compare yourself with someone else in the family or even one of your friends. Remember, cardiovascular endurance programs are individual in nature. What is good for one person may be inappropriate and even dangerous for another.

Part Three

The Battle of the Bulge:
Eating for Fitness

Probably no area of American life is clogged with so many fads and myths as nutrition and weight control. Someone reads the latest book on nutrition or dieting and becomes an instant expert on the subject. Americans have become known as the most overfed and undernourished people in the world. Television is a constant purveyor of the latest diets, the most "scientific" new equipment for losing weight in hours, the most exotic foods and drink. It is unusual to attend a social gathering where food is not served. We have become the most weight-conscious but nutritionally ignorant people in the civilized world.

Are you or any of the members of your family overweight? Chapter 5 will show you how to find out. You may be surprised to discover how easy it is to find out and even more surprised to discover what is really meant by overweight.

Do you think you know the best diet to lose or gain weight? You may be as confused as most people about proper dieting methods. You can find out in Chapter 6.

Chapter Five

Determining Recommended Body Weight

GOAL: Be able to administer and interpret body weight tests for yourself and any member of your family.

Your weight is not the best measure of whether or not you are overweight. Even standard height, weight, and age charts are of little help. Overweight is best judged on the basis of how much fat you carry in your body tissues. Typical weight scales don't tell you this. A weight gain may be the result of lean muscle mass increase or an increase in fat. Since it takes five times as much fat as lean muscle mass to equal one pound, however, even a slight increase in body weight can mean a significant increase in fat.

The best weight for you is the weight at which you feel your best. No scientist can predict the best weight for you or any other member of your family. A great deal of work is being done to establish charts that are based on percent body fat related to type of body frame. However, no one has yet decided how to determine one's body frame type. By the same token, no one has been able to determine the optimal percentage of body fat for a given individual. At the present time, we can only estimate that for maintenance of good health, percent body fat for males should range somewhere between 10 and 15 percent, while the range for females should be somewhere between 15 and 20 percent.

Body fat measurements can be direct and very accurate, such as underwater (hydrostatic) weighing or by chemical analysis (which can be done only on dead tissue). However, such measurements are not practical except in the laboratory. In spite of problems in determining the best weight for any individual, there are three simple tests you can use to

FIGURE 5-1
BODY WEIGHT FITNESS APPRAISAL

1. Name _Sharon Livewell_ _____Date _____
2. Current Weight _____135_____Sex ___F_____Age _34_____

Body Fat Test 1: Mirror Test

3. Look at yourself unclothed in a mirror. Are there bulges and loose, flabby skin in one or more of the following places: the mid-section, the buttocks, the thighs (especially behind the upper part of the legs)?

   Yes_____X_____(You are overfat) No_____(You are not overfat)

Body Fat Test 2: Pinch Test

4. Indicate whether or not you pinched one inch thick or more of skin in each of the following areas:

	Less than 1"	One inch or more
(a) side of the belly		X
(b) waist		X
(c) thigh		X
(d) buttocks		X
(e) back of the arm		X

5. Was the thickness of the skin at any one or more of the five points in Item 4 one inch thick or more?

   Yes___X_____(You are overfat) No_____(You are not overfat)
   Percent body fat_____30_____

Body Fat Test 3: Skinfold Caliper Test

6. Type of caliper used:
   Standard fat caliper_____Hand-controlled pressure caliper_____X_____

94

FIGURE 5-1 (continued)
BODY WEIGHT FITNESS APPRAISAL

7. Skinfolds as measured by caliper:

		1st Measure (mm)	2nd Measure (mm)	Average
(a)	iliac crest (top of hip)	17	18.5	17.8
(b)	triceps (back of upper arm)	17.5	17.5	17.5
(c)	biceps (front of upper arm)	6	7	6.5
(d)	subscapular (below shoulder blade)	8	8	8

8. Sum of averages of skin folds at four sites   49.8

9. Percent body fat   27.5

*Body fat content as indicated by sum of skinfolds at four sites**

	Fat as Percent of Body Weight			
Total Skinfold (mm)	Men	Women	Boys	Girls
15	5.5	— —	9.0	12.5
20	9.0	15.5	12.5	16.0
25	11.5	18.5	15.5	19.0
30	13.5	21.0	17.5	21.5
35	15.5	23.0	19.5	23.5
40	17.0	24.5	21.5	25.0
45	18.5	26.0	23.0	27.0
50	20.0	27.5	24.0	28.5
55	21.0	29.0	25.5	29.5
60	22.0	30.0	26.5	30.5
65	23.0	31.0	27.5	32.0
70	24.0	32.5	28.5	33.0
75	25.0	33.5	29.5	34.0
80	26.0	34.0		
85	26.5	35.0		
90	27.5	36.0		
95	28.0	36.5		

*Olaf Mickelsen, "Exercise and Weight Control" in *Physical Activity in Modern Living,* 2nd Edition, by Van Huss/Niemeyer/Olson/Friedrich, © 1969, pg. 157. Reprinted by permission of Prentice-Hall, Inc., Englewood Cliffs, New Jersey.

FIGURE 5-1 (continued)
BODY WEIGHT FITNESS APPRAISAL

10.	Current weight	135 ~~140~~
11.	Current percent body fat (from line 9)	X .28
12.	Total pounds of fat (line 11 *times* line 10)	38
13.	Current weight	135
*14.	Desired percent body fat (males 15%; female 20%)	X .20
15.	Desired pounds of fat (line 13 *times* line 14)	27
16.	Pounds to lose (line 12 *minus* line 15)	11
17.	Current weight	135
18.	Pounds to lose (from line 16)	-11
†19.	Target weight (line 17 *minus* line 18)	124

---

*This figure for women varies from 15 to 20 percent body fat and for men 10 to 15 percent body fat, depending on body build, amount of exercise, and the individual's own sense of "feeling good."

†This is only an estimate, especially if you engage in vigorous exercise. With exercise you may gain weight but lose fat because your muscles are becoming larger and stronger.

---

estimate whether or not a family member is ¨overfat.¨ The first test described in this chapter is the simplest, the mirror test. Only slightly more complicated is the pinch test. The most complicated of the three tests is the skinfold caliper test, which also allows you to estimate the best weight for yourself or any other family member. This test requires special equipment that need not be expensive.

When you learn how to administer and interpret these three tests, you will be able to do a far better job than the best of the height-weight charts in determining whether or not any family member is overfat, and what his or her recommended body weight is.

PROCEDURES

Each member of the family should fill out a separate body weight fitness appraisal form as the procedures in this chapter are followed. As these procedures are described, notice how Sharon Livewell's form is filled in (Figure 5-1). Remember, Sharon, the mother in the Livewell family, is concerned because she is gaining weight. Before you begin any of these tests, it is wise to have a thorough medical examination. Instructions relative to this medical examination are in Chapter 3.

Before beginning the body weight tests, fill in lines 1 and 2 on the body weight fitness appraisal, including the person's name and sex, the date of the tests, current weight (use a weight scale that will be used frequently by family members), and the person's age.

Body Fat Test 1: Mirror Test

Look at yourself unclothed in a mirror. If you look fat, you are fat — as simple as that. Notice particularly those areas where fat tends to show most: the mid-section, the buttocks, the thighs (especially behind the upper part of the legs). If the skin is loose and flabby, you are overfat. Indicate on line 3 whether or not you are overfat.

It wasn't difficult for Sharon Livewell to figure out she was overfat. She likes to eat and in spite of her activities as a homemaker, a PTA worker, and a hospital volunteer, she does not get enough exercise to rid herself of those extra calories. After looking at herself in the mirror, she checked yes on line 3 because she is overfat. The roll of flesh around her mid-section and the one beginning behind the upper part of her thighs were unmistakable indications that she was overfat.

Body Fat Test 2: Pinch Test

Find a book, a board, or a set of magazines exactly one inch thick.[1] Practice pinching it in one spot between your thumb and index finger until you get the feel for something one inch thick. Then, by applying pressure between these two fingers, pull away, lift, and pinch a fold of skin and underlying fat tissue from the muscle tissue below, using moderate pressure, in the following areas:

1. At the side of the belly
2. The waist
3. The thigh
4. The buttocks
5. The back of the arm

Indicate on the appropriate item for line 4 whether or not you pinched one inch or more. If the thickness of skin in any *one* of these five areas was one inch thick or more, mark yes on line 5 (meaning you are overfat). Other-

---

[1]Pinch test is adapted from L. E. Morehouse & L. Gross, *Total Fitness in 30 Minutes a Week* (New York: Simon and Schuster, 1975).

wise, mark no on line 5 (meaning you are not overfat). Sharon Livewell could pinch more than one inch at each of the five sites as indicated on line 4. Therefore, she marked yes on line 5, meaning she is overfat.

One inch of pinch amounts to about forty pounds of fat in the average adult. Every additional quarter inch means ten additional pounds of fat on the average. This means that you have a given number of pounds of fat in your total body weight. Remember, however, that you *should* have *some* fat in the body. Sharon has approximately forty pounds of fat in her body, because she could feel an inch of pinch at each of the designated places on her body. She can easily find out what percent of her body weight is fat by dividing the number of pounds of fat (40) by her weight (135). Sharon has approximately 30 percent body fat so she wrote that number on the percent body fat line for item 5. The ideal percent body fat for a woman is 15 to 20 percent, so Sharon knows she has some fat to lose.

Body Fat Test 3: Skinfold Caliper Test

The most accurate and practical test of your percent body fat is to use a skinfold caliper.[2] You will need the assistance of someone else to conduct this test. Hospital supply stores have standard fat calipers where pressure can be set and a reading taken directly from the caliper dial. However, these are beyond the budget of most people. Therefore, a small, hand-controlled pressure caliper can be purchased inexpensively at a hardware or craft store. Readings can be taken by measuring the distance between the two points on the caliper, using the millimeter scale on an ordinary ruler. This measure is less accurate than the special skinfold calipers but just as useful for all practical purposes.

On line 6 of the body weight fitness appraisal form, indicate the type of caliper used. If it is a special caliper used only for measuring body fat, mark standard fat caliper. If it is a hand-controlled pressure caliper purchased in a hardware or craft store, mark that space on line 6. Sharon Livewell used a hand-controlled pressure caliper she purchased in the local hardware store. Her husband, Michael, measured her skinfolds for this test.

The fingertips of the thumb and forefinger of one hand are used to lift the skin and fat up and away from underlying muscle tissue, using moderate pressure. If using a *standard skinfold caliper*, release the handle of the caliper to allow full force of the caliper arm pressure. A reading is made to the nearest .5 millimeter. When using a *hand-controlled pressure-operated caliper* (purchased in a hardware or a craft store), squeeze it to the

---

[2]Skinfold caliper test is adapted from F. Vitale, *Individualized Fitness Programs* (Englewood Cliffs, New Jersey: Prentice-Hall, 1973).

threshold of pain. Then measure with an ordinary ruler, using the millimeter reading on the ruler.

To insure as much accuracy as possible, take *two* skinfold applications at each of the four sites. If skinfolds are extremely thick (over one inch), take the reading three seconds after applying caliper pressure. Take the skinfold measurements in the morning soon after arising to avoid variations due to tissue dehydration. Take two measurements at each of these four sites and write the measures on lines 7a, 7b, 7c, and 7d as indicated:

Iliac crest (top of the hip) – Line 7a. Pick up a skinfold halfway between the lower rib and the hip bone in a vertical line extending from the armpit.

Triceps (back of the upper arm) – Line 7b. With the arm hanging loose alongside the body, take a skinfold on a vertical line halfway between the elbow and armpit.

Biceps (front of the upper arm) – Line 7c. Same as triceps measurements only on the front of the arm.

Subscapular (just below the lower part of the shoulder blade) – Line 7d. Pick up a skinfold just below the shoulder blade on the natural fold running parallel to the shoulder blade.

After two skinfold measurements have been taken at each of the four sites and the millimeter reading indicated on the appropriate lines of item 7 on the body weight fitness appraisal form, the next step is to take an average

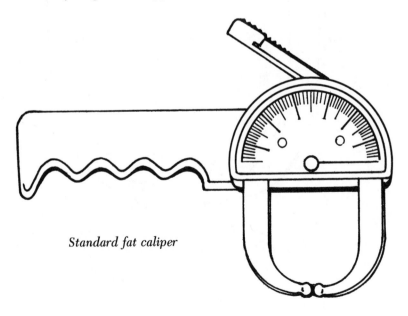

Standard fat caliper

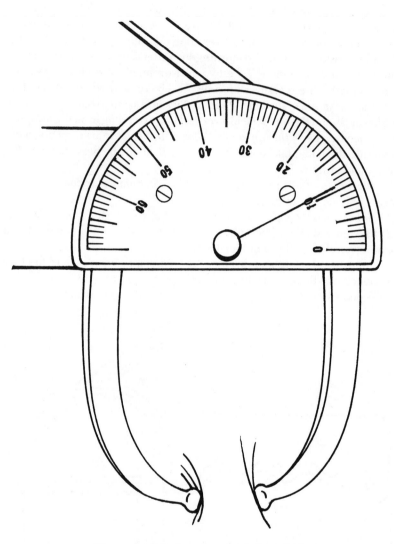

*Close-up of dial on standard fat caliper
as it pinches some skin*

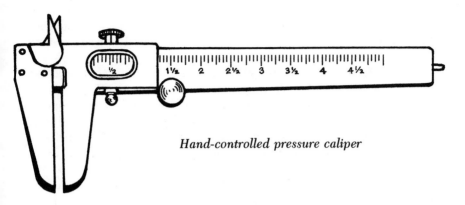

Hand-controlled pressure caliper

of the two measurements at each site and write that average in the third space for each site on the form. For instance, Sharon Livewell's first measure on her iliac crest above the hip (line 7a) was 17; the second measure was 18.5. The average of 17 and 18.5 is 17.8, so 17.8 is written on the third space at the far right on line 7a. The same thing was done for Sharon's triceps, biceps, and subscapular measurements.

The next step is to add up the averages of the four skinfold sites (line 8). In Sharon's case, the sum of all four averages was 49.8.

To find the percent body fat (line 90), go to the chart immediately following line 9. Using the sum from line 8, go to the left-hand column on the chart, Total Skinfold (mm). Find the number in this column that is nearest the sum from line 8. For Sharon, the sum from line 8, 49.8, is nearest 50 in the left-hand column. Since Sharon is a woman, she goes to the third column, Women, on the chart to find out her percent body fat (that is, the amount of her total body weight that is fat). Drawing her finger horizontally across the chart from 50 in the left-hand column to the corresponding number in the Women column, Sharon finds that she is 27.5 percent body fat, so she writes 27.5 on line 9. If the skinfold measurements are for a man, use the second column on the chart to find his percent body fat; if a boy, use the fourth column; if a girl, use the fifth column to find percent body fat. (Use the Boys and Girls columns for children twelve years of age and under.)

(*Note:* Generally women are considered obese if they have 27 percent or more of their total body weight in fat. For men, this is 20 percent or more. Since Sharon has 27.5 percent body fat, she is considered to be obese or overfat. Sharon's skinfold measurements are very close to the more general pinch test [27.5 vs. 30 percent].)

Once you have estimated your percent body fat using the Skinfold

Caliper Test, you may wish to find out how many pounds of fat you have, how many pounds you need to lose, and what your target weight should be. Lines 10 through 20 on the body weight fitness appraisal form allow you to do this.

Line 10. Write on line 10 your current weight. This is the same as the weight you wrote on line 2. Sharon Livewell's weight is 135.

Line 11. Write on line 11 your current percent body fat from line 9. Put the decimal in the correct place because you will be multiplying. Sharon's current percent body fat is 28 percent (the next higher percent from 27.5 so she won't need to deal in half percents), so she writes .28 on line 11.

Line 12. In order to find out how many pounds of fat you have in your body, multiply your current weight (line 10) by your current percent body fat (line 11). Round off your answer to the nearest pound and write it on line 12. Sharon multiplied her current weight on line 10 (135) by her current percent body fat on line 11 (.28) and arrived at a figure of 38 pounds of fat on line 12.

Line 13. Write your current weight again, this time on line 13, because you are now going to figure how many pounds you may need to lose. In order to do this, you need to include your current weight in the arithmetic again.

Line 14. On line 14 write your desired percent body fat. For males this can vary from 10 to 15 percent; for females, from 15 to 20 percent. This desired percent depends upon your body build, the amount of exercise you get, and your own sense of "feeling good." Since you really don't know yet what your best percent body fat is, the best estimate to use is the maximum estimate. Thus, if you are male, write .15 on line 14. If you are female, write .20. Sharon is a female, so she wrote .20 on line 14.

Line 15. Now you are ready to find the desired pounds of fat for your own body. In order to do this, simply multiply your current weight (line 13) by your desired percent body fat (line 14). Round off your answer to the nearest pound and write it on line 15. Sharon multiplied her current weight on line 13 (135) by her desired percent body fat on line 14 (.20) and arrived at a figure of 27 desired pounds of fat on line 15.

Line 16. Now it is a simple matter to figure out how many pounds you may need to lose. Simply subtract from your total pounds of fat on line 12 the desired pounds of fat on line 15. Put your answer on line 16. Sharon subtracted from her total pounds of fat on line 12 (38) the desired pounds of fat on line 15 (27) and found she had 11 pounds to lose, which she wrote on line 16.

Line 17. This is the last time you need to write your current weight. You need it this time to figure what your target weight is (that is, how much you should weigh if you lose the number of pounds you indicated on line 16). Sharon again wrote 135.

Line 18. Now write on line 18 the number of pounds you need to lose (from line 16). Sharon wrote 11.

Line 19. Now you are ready to find a pretty good estimate of how much you should weigh — your target weight. Simply subtract from your current weight (line 17) the pounds you need to lose (line 18). Write your answer on line 19. Sharon subtracted from her current weight on line 17 (135) the number of pounds she needs to lose on line 18 (11) and found her target weight is 124 (line 19). Your target weight is only an estimate, especially if you engage frequently in vigorous exercise. With exercise you may gain weight but lose fat because your muscles are becoming larger and stronger.

Remember, all these tests are estimates only. Your best guideline is the way you feel.

Chapter Six

Planning a Weight Control Program

GOAL: Be able to plan a weight control program for yourself or any other member of your family.

No matter how magazine articles or newspapers try to make the idea of being overweight a little more palatable for the public, the fact remains that fat accumulates in the body when you eat more calories than your body uses. That is, if you eat food containing 2700 calories a day and your body uses only 2400 calories a day, your body has 300 extra calories a day. This is stored as fat. There are 3500 calories in one pound of fat. At that rate of calorie intake and usage, you would gain one pound every twelve days.

In Chapter 5, you learned how to find out if you are overfat and what your ideal weight should be. In this chapter you will learn how to plan a daily diet that is both nutritious and low in calories to help you achieve, gradually, your ideal weight. The emphasis is on a *gradual* reduction in weight — no more than one pound per week. If you have more than forty pounds to lose to achieve your ideal weight, it would probably be a good idea to have your physician help plan your diet. Physicians occasionally will have their patients go on a diet of less than 1200 calories a day, which means you must miss some basic nutrients in your daily diet. That is why such a diet should be planned and engaged in only under the close supervision of a physician. The rule for this chapter, and for any good weight control program over a long period of time, is this: *Eat a fully nutritious diet each day.*

Here are the basic requirements of a successful weight-loss program:
1. The daily diet should include fewer calories than the body uses for

energy each day. That is, there should be a daily calorie deficit. This means the body will use excess fat already stored in the body to meet its complete energy needs.

2. The daily diet should be nutritious. That is, it should meet the body's needs for proteins, carbohydrates, fats, vitamins, minerals, and trace elements. These needs are met when foods are selected from a variety of foods in each of the four basic food groups: the milk group, the meat group, the vegetable and fruit group, the bread and cereal group.

3. The diet, when followed, should produce a gradual weight loss. If the weight loss is dramatic, the loss of weight is probably caused by loss of lean body tissue, not fatty tissue. It is also likely that the body's nutrient needs are not being met. Such weight is quickly regained.

4. An important component of the reducing program is an exercise program. Unless a proper exercise program accompanies a reducing diet, weight loss will include lean body tissue as well as fatty tissue. When exercise (see Parts One and Two of this book) is included, most of the weight loss will be fatty tissue. At the same time, the muscles of the body will be stronger, more flexible, and in better working condition. In other words, you will feel better in spite of a lower intake of calories.

5. The reducing plan should be flexible enough to be adapted to a lifetime of use. Therefore, the eating habits you develop in a reducing plan should be a part of your daily diet throughout your lifetime. The needed adjustments will include only amounts of food, not types of food.

At the end of this chapter you will find a series of frequently asked questions and answers about weight control. Now we look at how to plan a weight control program, focusing on weight reduction.

PROCEDURES

There are six basic steps to any effective weight control program for any member of the family:

1. Determine how many calories you are presently eating each day.
2. Determine your daily calorie intake in order to lose one pound a week.
3. Find the appropriate daily food plan.
4. Implement the daily food plan.
5. Record daily weight.
6. Reward yourself for sticking to your diet.

STEP 1: *Determine How Many Calories You Are Presently Eating Each Day*

FIGURE 6-1
FOOD INTAKE RECORD

Name Sharon Livewell

Date	Description of Food Item	Amount		Calories
9/15	Toast	2 slices	(68)	136
	Butter (on toast)	2 tsp.	(45)	90
	Milk (whole)	2 cups	(170)	340
	Cheese sandwich	1 slice bread		68
		2 slices cheese	(73)	146
	Tamale pie	1 cup		68+146=214
				(corn + meat)
	Green beans	1 cup		---
	Butter (on beans)	1 tsp.		45
	Bread	1 slice		68
	Butter (on bread)	1 tsp.		45
	Ice cream	1 cup		136
	Pop corn	3 cups		136
	Butter (on pop corn)	1 tbs.	(45)	135
	Daily Total			1559
9/16	Canned cherries	1 cup	(40)	80
	Sugar (in cherries)	2 tsp.	(16)	32
	Peanut butter sandwich	2 slices bread	(68)	136
	Peanut butter	2 tbs.		73
	Orange juice	1 cup	(40)	80
	Stuffed pork chop	6 oz.	(73x6)	438
	Green salad	1½ cups		---
	Salad dressing	1 tbs.	(45x3)	135
	Peas	½ cup		36
	Corn	⅓ cup		68
	Cookie	1 medium		50
	Jello	1 cup	(68x2)	136
	Cinnamon roll	1 medium		176
	Daily Total			1440
9/17	Banana	1 whole	(40x2)	80
	Orange	1 medium		40
	Tomato soup	1 cup		36
	Root beer	1 cup		40
	Fish	6 oz.	(73x6)	438
	Bread	2 slices	(68x2)	136
	Butter (on bread)	2 tsp.	(45x2)	90
	Cheese	2 slices	(73x2)	146
	Milk (whole)	1 cup		170
	Cinnamon roll	2 medium	(176x2)	352
	Daily Total			1528
	Three-day Grand Total			4527
	Average Daily Calories			1509

107

FIGURE 6-2
FOOD EXCHANGE LIST

Meat Exchange List
Each exchange = 73 calories

FOOD	MEASURE
Cheese	
American, Cheddar, Swiss	1 oz., 1 slice, 1" cube, or ¼ cup grated
Cottage, not creamed	¼ cup
Cold cuts (bologna, braunschweiger, luncheon loaf, minced ham, salami, cotto)	1 oz. = 1 slice (4½" diameter, ⅛" thick)
Eggs	1
Fish	
Cod, halibut, haddock, trout, snapper, etc. (cooked)	1 oz.
Crabmeat, lobster	¼ cup
Sardines	3 medium
Shrimp, clams, oysters	5 small
Tuna, salmon	¼ cup
Frankfurter	1
Meat, poultry (no bone or visible fat) (beef, chicken, corned beef, ham, lamb, liver, pork, turkey, veal)	1 oz. cooked or 3½" X 2" X ¼"
Peanut butter	2 tbs.

Milk Exchange List
Each exchange = 170 calories

FOOD	MEASURE
Milk, whole	1 cup
Milk, 2% butterfat*	1 cup
Milk, skim or fat-free†	1 cup
Dried whole milk powder†	¼ cup
Dried skim milk powder†	¼ cup
Evaporated milk	½ cup
Evaporated skim milk†	½ cup
Buttermilk made from skim milk	1 cup
Plain yogurt	1 cup

*Add 1 fat exchange to diet
†Add 2 fat exchanges to diet

Fruit Exchange List
Each exchange = 40 calories

FOOD	MEASURE
Apple	1 small (2" diam.)
Apple juice	⅓ cup
Applesauce	½ cup
Apricots, fresh	2 medium
Apricots, dried	4 halves

FOOD EXCHANGE LIST (Continued)

Apricots, canned (unsweetened)	1/2 cup
Apricot nectar	1/3 cup
Banana	1/2 small
Berries (blackberries, raspberries, strawberries)	1 cup
Blueberries	2/3 cup
Cantaloupe	1/4 (6" diam.)
Cherries, fresh	10 large
Cherries, canned (unsweetened)	1/2 cup
Cranberry juice cocktail, canned	1/4 cup
Dates	2
Figs, fresh or dried	1
Grapefruit	1/2 small
Grapefruit juice	1/2 cup
Grapes	12
Grape juice	1/4 cup
Honeydew melon	1/8 (7" diam.)
Mango	1/2 small
Nectarine	1 medium
Orange	1 small
Orange juice	1/2 cup
Papaya	1/3 medium
Peach	1 medium
Peach, canned (unsweetened)	1/2 cup or 2 halves
Pear	1 small
Pear, canned (unsweetened)	1/2 cup or 2 halves
Pineapple, canned (unsweetened)	1/2 cup or 2 small slices
Plums	2 medium
Pomegranates	1 small
Prunes, dried	2
Prune juice	1/4 cup
Raisins	2 tbs.
Tangerine	1 large
Watermelon	1 cup or 1/2 slice, 3/4" thick

Vegetable Exchange Lists

A *Vegetables* (negligible caloric value). May be eaten in unlimited amounts if uncooked. If cooked, limit the amount eaten to one cup per day. When desired, an additional cup of A vegetable may be eaten in place of a B vegetable exchange.

Asparagus	*Escarole
Bean sprouts	*Greens
Beans, green or wax	Beet greens
°*Broccoli	Chard
°Brussel sprouts	Collards
°Cabbage	Dandelion
°Cauliflower	Kale
Celery	Mustard
*Chicory	Poke
Cucumbers	Spinach
Eggplant	Endive
Lettuce	Turnip greens
	Rhubarb

109

FIGURE 6-2
FOOD EXCHANGE LIST (Continued)

Mushrooms
Okra
Parsley
°Peppers
Pimento
Radishes
Romaine
Sauerkraut

Squash, summer (zucchini, gooseneck)
°Tomatoes
Tomato juice
Vegetable juice
*Watercress

B Vegetables

Each exchange = 36 calories

Artichoke (½ medium)
Beets
*Carrots
Peas, green
*Pumpkin

Rutabagas
°Squash, winter (butternut, acorn)
Turnips

*These vegetables are good sources of Vitamin C. At least one good source of Vitamin C should be eaten each day.

° These vegetables are good sources of Vitamin A. A good source of Vitamin A should be eaten at least every other day.

Bread and Cereal Exchange List
Each exchange = 68 calories

FOOD	MEASURE
Breads and Cereals	
Biscuit	2" diameter
Bread, baker's	1 slice
Cereals, cooked	½ cup
Cereals, dry (flakes or puffed, no sugar added)	¾ cup
Cornbread	1½" cube
Cornstarch	2 tbs.
Cracker meal	3 tbs.
Flour	3 tbs.
Grits, cooked	½ cup
Hamburger bun	1 small
Hot dog bun	1 small
Macaroni, noodles, spaghetti, cooked	½ cup
Muffin	2" diameter
Pancake	4" diameter
Rice	½ cup
Tortilla	6" diameter
Waffle	4" diameter

FIGURE 6-2
FOOD EXCHANGE LIST (Continued)

Sherbet	⅓ cup
Wheat wafers	7

Crackers	
Graham	2 squares
Oyster	20 (½ cup)
Saltines	5
Soda	3
Round, thin varieties	6-8

Vegetables

Beans, peas, dried (cooked) Includes: limas, navy, kidney beans; black-eyed (cowpeas), split, etc.	¼ cup
Baked beans, no pork	½ cup
Corn, cooked	⅓ cup
Corn on the cob	½ ear
Parsnips	½ cup
Potato, white baked	2″ diameter
Potatoes, white mashed	½ cup
Potato, sweet, or yams	¼ cup

Miscellaneous

Angel food cake	1½″ cube
Ice cream (omit 2 fat exchanges)	½ cup
Ice cream cone (not sugar cone, without ice cream)	1 cone
Popcorn (without butter)	1½ cup
3-ring pretzels	6

Fat Exchange List
Each exchange = 45 calories

FOOD	MEASURE
Avocado	⅛ (4″ diameter)
Butter or margarine	1 tsp.
Bacon	1 slice
Cream, light	2 tbs.
Cream, sour	2 tbs.
Cream, whipping	1 tbs.
Cream cheese	1 tbs.
Mayonnaise	1 tsp.
Oil or cooking fat	1 tsp.
Olives	5 small
Nuts	6 small
Shortening	1 tsp.
Tartar sauce	2 tsp.
Salad dressings (blue cheese, French, Italian, thousand island, etc.)	1 tbs.

FIGURE 6-2
FOOD EXCHANGE LIST (Continued)

Free List

The following foods are low in caloric content and may be eaten as desired.

Broth, fat free
Bouillon
Carbonated beverages, low-calorie (less than 5 calories per bottle)
Catsup (1 tsp.)
Chili sauce (1 tsp.)
Consommé
Cranberries, unsweetened
Gelatin, unflavored or artificially sweetened
Horseradish
Hot sauce
Jams and jellies that are artificially sweetened, low-calorie
Lemon juice
Mustard, prepared
Pickles, sour or dill
Rennet tablets
Salad dressings, low-calorie (less than 5 calories per tbs.)
Seasonings and spices (cinnamon, basil, celery salt, garlic, mint, mustard, nutmeg, oregano, parsley, pepper, etc.)

Sweeteners, low-calorie (saccharin, Sugar Twin, etc.)
Vanilla
Vinegar

Sweets

FOOD	MEASURE	CALORIES
Sugar, granulated	1 tbs.	48
Sugar, granulated	1 tsp.	16
Sugar, granulated	1 cup	770
Honey	1 tbs.	67
Jam	1 tbs.	58
Corn syrup	1 tbs.	59
Soda pop	1 cup	40
Sweet roll	medium	176
Cookie	medium	50
Hard candy	average piece	29
Chocolate syrup	1 tbs.	48

Commercially Prepared Exchanges

This list may be used in applying some commercially prepared products to the exchange lists.

Dessert topping mix, low-calorie, prepared according to package directions; 1/3 cup = 1 fat exchange

112

FIGURE 6-2
FOOD EXCHANGE LIST (Continued)

Fish sticks, frozen; 3-1 oz. sticks = ½ bread exchange and 2 meat exchanges

Gelatin, flavored, sweetened, ready to eat; ½ cup = 1 bread exchange

Mayonnaise, low-calorie; 2 tbs. = 1 fat exchange

Tomato paste, 3 tbs. = 1 B vegetable exchange

Tomato sauce, ¼ cup = 1 B vegetable exchange and 1 fat exchange

Soups (values are given for ½ can of condensed soup before water or milk is added)

Beef = ½ meat exchange and ½ vegetable exchange

Beef noodle = ½ meat exchange and 1 bread exchange

Black bean = 2 bread exchanges

Bouillon = free

Chicken gumbo = ½ bread exchange and ½ fat exchange

Chicken noodle = 1 bread exchange

Chicken rice = ½ meat exchange and ½ bread exchange

Chicken vegetable = 1 bread exchange and ½ fat exchange

Clam chowder; Manhattan style = 1 bread exchange and ½ fat exchange

Clear broth = free

Consommé = free

Cream of asparagus = ½ vegetable exchange and ½ fat exchange

Cream of celery = ½ vegetable exchange and ½ fat exchange

Cream of chicken = ½ vegetable exchange and ½ fat exchange

Cream of mushroom = ½ vegetable exchange and 1 fat exchange

Cream of potato = vegetable exchange and ½ fat exchange

Green pea = 2½ bread exchanges

Minestrone = ½ vegetable exchange and 1 fat exchange

Onion soup = ½ vegetable exchange and ½ fat exchange

Pepper pot = ½ vegetable exchange and ½ fat exchange

Scotch broth = ½ meat exchange and ½ fat exchange

Tomato = 1 vegetable exchange

Turkey noodle = ½ meat exchange and ½ bread exchange

Vegetable = 1 vegetable exchange

Vegetable beef = ½ meat exchange and ½ vegetable exchange

Vegetarian vegetable = 1 vegetable exchange

Prater, Barbara M., Denton, Nancy J., and Oakeson, Kathleen. *Food and You*. Published by the authors, 1970. Reprinted by permission.

In order to develop a tailor-made weight control program for you or any family member, you must find out what your *present* food intake is. When you know what your present intake is, then it is possible to determine how much you should eliminate from your diet in order to lose weight. Keep a food intake record (see Figure 6-1) of what you ate during each of three days. Write the approximate amount of each food item eaten (in cups, half cups, tablespoons, etc.). At the end of each day look at the food exchange lists (Figure 6-2) and write the amount of calories for each food you ate that day. Then add up the total calories you ate that day.

After you have recorded what you eat for three days, add the three daily totals and divide this grand total by three. This will give you the average number of calories you now eat each day. This is the basic calorie total from which your weight control program can be figured.

Figure 6-1 shows Sharon Livewell's food intake record for three days. Her first item on the food intake record is toast. Since toast is a bread, she went to the bread exchange list on the food exchange list. She looked at the number of calories per serving at the beginning of the bread list, noting it was 68, meaning every item on the list had 68 calories. She found that one slice of bread is 68 calories. Since toast is considered a slice of bread, and she had two pieces of toast, Sharon wrote 136 in the calories column. She followed this procedure for each item she ate during that day. She estimated that she ate one teaspoon of butter on each slice of toast, so she looked in the fat exchange list for the number of calories. She had butter again later in the day on her green beans, so she made sure she included that additional teaspoon of butter. Tamale pie consists mainly of hamburger and corn and corn meal. She estimated one-third cup corn total (on the bread exchange list = 68 calories) and two ounces of hamburger (one ounce = 73 calories on meat exchange list) in the tamale pie for a total of 214 calories. By noting ingredients in various food items, she was able to figure out how many calories were in each food she ate each of the three days. At the end of each day she added the calorie list to get her daily calorie total (1559 on the first day, 1440 on the second day, and 1528 on the third day). Then she added the three daily totals to get a grand total for three days (4527). She divided the grand total by three and arrived at an average daily calorie intake of 1509 (this can be rounded off to the nearest 100, or 1500 in this case). Now Sharon is ready to move to the next step.

STEP 2: *Determine Your Daily Calorie Intake in Order to Lose One Pound a Week*

One pound of fat is equivalent to 3500 calories. In order to lose one pound each week, you must lower your weekly calorie intake by 3500 calories, or 500 calories each day (3500 calories divided by seven days =

FIGURE 6-3
DAILY FOOD PLANS

TYPE OF FOOD	DAILY CALORIE INTAKE													
	1200	1300	1400	1500	1600	1700	1800	1900	2000	2100	2200	2300	2400	2500
Vegetables*	1	1	1	1	1	1	2	2	2	2	2	2	2	2
Breads	4	4	5	5	6	6	6	7	7½	7½	9	10	10	10
Meats	5	5	6	6	6	6	7	7	8	8	8	8	9	9
Milk	2	2	2	2	2	2½	2½	2½	2½	2½	2½	2½	2½	3
Fruits	4	4	3	4	4	4	4	5	5	6	6	6	6	6
Fats	1	3	3	4	5	5	5	5	5	6	6	7	7	8

*Numbers refer to servings of B vegetables in the food selection guide. A vegetables can be eaten in addition if you follow the guidelines for the vegetable exchange list in the food selection guide.

Note: If your daily food plan requires more than 2500 calories, you can still use these daily food plans. For instance, if your diet is for 2800 calories, just double the food plan for 1400 calories. For a 3000 calorie food plan, double the 1500 calorie list.

Adapted from "Meal Planning with Exchange Lists" developed by committees of the American Dietetic Association and the American Diabetes Association in cooperation with the Chronic Disease Program of the United States Public Health Service.

500 calories). If your daily calorie intake in Step 1 was 2400 calories, you would need to subtract 500 calories a day from 2400 in order to lose one pound a week. This means your daily calorie intake should be 1900 calories instead of the usual 2400 if you wish to lose weight. If your daily intake in Step 1 was 2150 calories, your daily calorie intake should be 1600 calories (1650 rounded off to the next lowest 100).

Inasmuch as Sharon Livewell found out she was eating 1500 calories a day, she must reduce her daily calorie intake to 1000 (500 subtracted from 1500) in order to lose one pound per week. It is not wise to eat fewer than 1200 calories a day without the supervision of a physician. Therefore, Sharon decided her daily calorie intake should be 1200 calories.

STEP 3: *Find the Appropriate Daily Food Plan*

We have emphasized the importance of including in your daily food intake all the necessary nutrients for good health. We have made this easy for you. Once you have determined what your daily calorie intake should be, go to the daily food plans chart (Figure 6-3) and find the column (to the next lowest 100) that show your daily calorie intake. This column tells you how many servings of each of the basic foods (vegetables, breads, meats, milk, fruits, fats) you can have each day. If your daily calorie intake should be 1400 calories, go to the third column from the left on the daily food plans chart. This indicates that you can have one serving of vegetables, five

FIGURE 6-4
CALORIE CARD

	1200 Calories	Date_____
Vegetables ____		
Breads ____ ____ ____ ____		
Meats ____ ____ ____ ____ ____		
Milks ____ ____		
Fruits ____ ____ ____ ____		
Fats ____		

breads, six meats, two milk, three fruits, and three fats. The measuring of these servings will be explained in the next step.

Sharon Livewell's daily calorie intake should be 1200 calories. She went to the column 1200 on the daily food plans chart and found out she could have one serving of vegetables, four breads, five meats, two milks, four fruits, and one fat. In order to make it easy for her to keep track of her daily food intake she made some cards that listed the food types down the left side of the card. The number of servings allowed for each food was indicated by the number of blanks at the side of each food type. Figure 6-4 shows a sample card for Sharon. All Sharon has to do is check off each food serving she eats during the day in the appropriate blank. When all the blanks are filled, she has eaten her quota of calories for the day.

STEP 4: *Implement the Daily Food Plan*

Once you have determined your food plan to lose one pound each week (and have made cards to keep track of what you eat), it is time to put the food plan into practice. This means you can go to the food exchange list to find out how much you can have of each kind of food on your food plan.

You will have to determine for yourself how you will divide up the foods you eat for each of the three meals. If your food plan allows you five breads daily, you won't want to eat all five servings of bread at one meal.

You may wish to have cereal (one bread) for breakfast, a sandwich for lunch (two breads) and a medium potato for dinner (two breads). You would do the same kind of planning for the other foods on your food plan.

Exact measurements are very important. Avoid estimating. If the food exchange list says one serving is one-half cup of a food item, measure exactly one-half cup. If one serving is one ounce of a food item, weigh one ounce on a food scale. (Food scales can be purchased inexpensively at most variety or housewares stores.)

Eat *three meals a day.* Don't starve all day and then eat everything in your food plan at the evening meal. The body needs time to handle the food you eat. If you gorge yourself, you are defeating your weight loss program because the body will convert much of what you "overeat" as fat, simply because it will use only what it needs at the present time for nutrients and energy and store the rest in the form of fat. In other words, weight loss is dependent not only on how many calories you eat, but when you eat those calories, and how many calories are eaten at one serving. Don't forget to check off on your daily food plan cards the foods you eat each day.

It is hoped you are also engaging in a vigorous and consistent exercise program. Don't add calories to your daily diet to make up for the energy you exert in exercise. Allow your exercise to be that "something extra" that may help you lose weight a little faster. The diet program suggested in this chapter is for an average weight loss of one pound per week. With exercise you may find yourself losing up to two pounds per week. It is not recommended that you attempt to lose weight any faster.

STEP 5: *Record Daily Weight*

When you start your weight control program, it's a good idea to keep a daily record of your weight. This daily record will help you see over time how your weight-loss program is progressing. Expect some slight fluctuations up and down the weight scale. These fluctuations are natural and should be of no concern.

At the beginning of your weight-loss program, you may not notice any weight loss at all for a week or ten days. Don't be discouraged. This is natural as the body tends to hold water while it adjusts to a slightly reduced daily food intake.

Remember, it took you a while to gain those pounds. Don't try to lose them all at once. Resist the urge to go on a crash diet to prepare for a special occasion, such as a posh dinner party or the visit of friends or relatives who have never seen you so heavy.

A daily weight record is provided for you to use in recording your daily weight. Figure 6-5 shows Sharon Livewell's daily weight record. Note the fluctuations on the chart but also the trend downward. Because Sharon was also engaging regularly in a cardiovascular exercise program (jogging) with her family, the calories she burned during exercise were an added burning of calories each day. Thus, her exercise helped to burn the extra calories she needed to get rid of each day.

Notice in Figure 6-5 that Sharon wrote in the weight figures on her daily weight record down the outer left column, beginning at the bottom a few pounds less than what she wanted to lose (her target weight is 124 pounds). She then wrote the number of pounds up the left side by one-pound increments until she had written a few pounds over her present weight (135). She wrote the dates across the bottom of the chart, beginning with the date she started her weight-loss program. Sharon's weight averaged about the same for the first ten days but then showed a steady but gradual trend downward. Such gradual loss of weight is easier to maintain at the end of the weight-loss period than is a sudden and dramatic weight loss.

If you have a willpower problem, it might be a good idea to post your daily weight record where the whole family can see it, such as on the refrigerator door. (Posting it on the refrigerator door also reminds you about your weight loss and can make it easier to avoid those calorie-rich refrigerator snacks.) This will give family members a chance to note your

Name: Sharon Livewell

FIGURE 6-5
DAILY WEIGHT RECORD

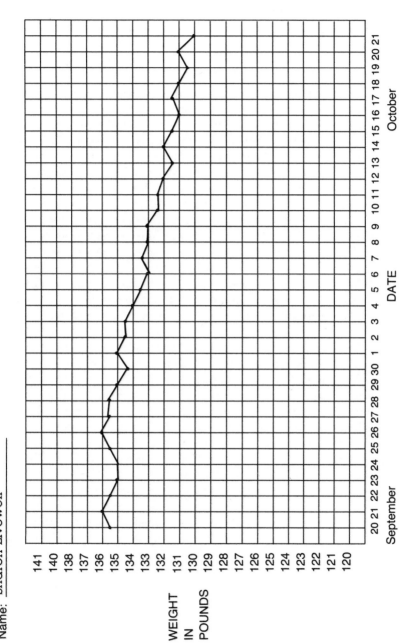

progress and give you a pat on the back for your efforts. It also is a good way to publicly commit yourself to a weight-loss program. When other people know what you plan to do and how you plan to do it, you are more likely to stick to your plan.

STEP 6: *Reward Yourself for Sticking to Your Diet*

Weight loss itself is such a strong reinforcer that you may not need any additional rewards for reducing your calorie intake. However, it generally is a good idea to plan some rewards for yourself along the way, just to keep up your incentive. Perhaps a movie or a sports event or a weekend trip contingent on your consistency in sticking to your diet will keep you going. The important rule is to make reward dependent on sticking to your daily food plan. If you will get the reward whether or not you stick to your diet, then it will not really be a reward for good eating habits.

In addition to occasional rewards during your weight-loss program, it might be wise to plan a large reward when you reach your target weight, such as a vacation trip to a special destination or a new outfit (or even a new wardrobe). Whatever you plan for rewards, they should be unique to *you*. What is rewarding to one person may be no incentive at all to another person. And by no means allow food to be a reward!

If you find after two or three weeks on this plan that you are not losing weight, it may be necessary for you to reduce your caloric intake by another 500 calories per day. For example, if your daily food plan was 1800 calories, you may need to reduce it to 1300 calories. It may take a little trial and error before you find a daily food plan that will allow you to lose one pound a week. Again, don't overdo it by saying to yourself, "If it is good to reduce my daily calorie intake by 500 calories, then reducing it by 1000 or 1500 calories would be better." Remember, if you lose weight too fast (that is, more than two pounds per week), you are losing primarily lean body tissue, not fatty tissue. This means you will gain it back hurriedly. The idea is to lose excess *fat*, not just excess weight.

Once you have reached your desired target weight, you can gradually increase your daily calorie intake in order to *maintain* your weight. This means you probably will need to permanently change your old eating habits so that you do not begin taking in extra calories that eventually add up to excess fat.

It is not necessary to go on a separate menu from the rest of the family when losing weight. The entire family's daily menus should be selected from the basic four food groups. The only difference between your daily food intake and that of other family members should be the amounts of each food you eat each day. The old adage that the best weight-loss exercise is pushing yourself away from the table is good only if you have partaken of the *right kinds* and *right amounts* of food while at the table. *Do not* skip meals.

Special Dieting Suggestions

1. Eat slowly. Chew every mouthful of food slowly, savoring the flavor as you chew and swallow.
2. Lay the fork or spoon down between each bite. People often tend to prepare the next bite on the utensil while chewing the preceding one. As a result, food often gets swallowed before it has been thoroughly chewed.
3. Save part of each meal for a snack later. This will prevent your being overhungry at mealtime. When you are ravenous, you tend to over-eat.
4. Serve yourself on smaller dishes — a salad or dessert plate instead of a dinner plate.
5. Include your favorite foods in your diet. If you like pie or cake, simply take smaller portions. You don't need to be an ascetic to diet successfully.
6. Prepare your foods in the most nutritious way with as few additional calories as possible. Avoid fried foods: broil, bake, boil, or roast meat and other vegetables. The new cooking bags for oven cooking retain moisture, nutrition, and flavor — and make food preparation very simple and easy. Eat vegetables raw when possible (*without* sugar). When cooking vegetables, steam them on low heat for as short a time as possible (add a pinch of sugar and salt to steamed or boiled vegetables to bring out the flavor). Eat raw fruits without sugar.
7. Weigh yourself consistently. Use the same scales. Wear the same clothing (or no clothing at all) each time you weigh yourself. Weigh yourself at the same time of day. Record your weight immediately each time you weigh yourself. Do not be discouraged if you don't lose weight the first week or two; this is normal but will change if you stick to your diet.

Avoid this weight-loss program if:

1. You are under pressure or emotional strain because of problems with school, spouse, boyfriend or girlfriend, job, finances, and so forth. If possible, get the problems solved before starting a weight-loss program.

2. You are unwilling to eat smaller amounts of food items than other family members.

3. You feel you cannot afford to purchase the types of foods necessary to maintain a balanced diet. It takes planning but can be relatively inexpensive to purchase less expensive brands and products.

4. You expect to lose a great deal of weight in a short period of time.

5.   You are unwilling to keep daily records of your weight and what you eat.

6.   Food is such an overwhelming reinforcer for you that you simply cannot replace food rewards with some other form of reward.

7.   You plan to go *off* your daily food plan and have occasional food binges (such as every weekend).

FREQUENTLY ASKED QUESTIONS

The first ten questions focus on the child in the family because nutrition problems in the home begin in childhood. Questions 11 through 30 are especially related to adults.

1.   *Is it possible for a child to drink too much milk?*

If a child drinks more than a quart of milk a day, he may be too full to eat foods that have other important nutrients milk does not contain, notably iron and Vitamin C.

2.   *How do you get a child to drink the milk he needs when he doesn't like milk?*

Pressure and even force from adults who are concerned about a child's milk consumption can turn him against milk. In such cases, it is a good idea to relax the pressure and make milk easily available for the child when he wants it. Most children enjoy milk when it is quite cold and served in a small glass or even another container, such as a colored cup or mug. Adding an occasional straw adds to the interest in drinking milk. If a child absolutely will not drink milk even when the pressure is off and you have tried everything else, use some ingenuity in the kitchen. Cook dishes that contain large amounts of milk such as milk-base soups (tomato or potato soups), chicken a la king, creamed vegetables, custards, ice cream, and puddings.

3.   *Is it better for children to eat margarine rather than butter?*

Butter is a good source of Vitamin A. Margarine does not have Vitamin A naturally. However, Vitamin A is now added to all margarines, making it almost equivalent in Vitamin A to butter. The fatty-acid composition of butter and margarine is very different. Butter has more highly concentrated fatty acids, whereas margarine has a higher percentage of polyunsaturated fatty acids. Thus margarine is easier to spread and more plastic than butter. The effect of highly concentrated vs. polyunsaturated fatty acids in the body is still controversial. At the present time, the best answer to this question seems to be that either butter or margarine may be eaten by children.

4.   *Is skim milk suitable for children to drink?*

Skim milk has had the fat removed and, thus, the Vitamin A and other fat-soluble vitamins. However, it is fortified with Vitamin D and is of a higher protein content than whole milk. Skim milk is just as suitable for a child's consumption as whole milk, especially if the child is overfat and needs a daily reduction of calorie intake. When skim milk is used consistently, however, care should be taken to insure Vitamin A intake from other foods.

5. *Should children eat candy?*

Ideally, the answer is no because of the effect of sugar on teeth. However, it is unrealistic to protect children from candy. If parents do not make candy available in the home, it is unlikely the candy eaten by children as treats elsewhere, such as when visiting grandparents, will be excessive.

6. *Should children drink carbonated drinks and sugar-flavored fruit drinks?*

Again, the ideal answer is no because of the sugar content. Also, where there is a high expenditure in the food budget for such drinks, there is usually a deficiency in the budget — and in the diet — for food items with proper nutrition. The problem becomes more intense during hot weather when there is a high intake of liquids. It is best to keep naturally sweetened fruit juices in the refrigerator for such purposes. For variety, children enjoy popsicles and ice cubes made from naturally flavored fruit juices, either fresh, frozen, or canned. The average American consumes 150 pounds of sugar and 15 pounds of corn syrup per year. This is a ridiculous amount, undoubtedly contributing to the incidence of more health problems than just dental caries. The high consumption of carbonated and sugar-flavored fruit drinks is a large part of this high sugar consumption. It should be discouraged in children, but adults need to set the example.

7. *Is it better for children to eat iodized salt or plain salt?*

If a person does not consume iodine, his thyroid gland enlarges gradually in a futile attempt to produce enough thyroxine for the body. This enlargement is called "endemic goiter." Iodine has been added to salt to provide the needed iodine in the diet because the only other source is saltwater fish. Saltwater fish is not available in adequate amounts in many parts of the country. Therefore, iodized salt is the means of obtaining needed iodine for the body. Although iodized salt is sold side by side with plain salt in the stores, many people buy plain salt because they do not understand the need for iodine. It is better that children eat iodized salt in their food.

8. *Should children receive vitamin supplements?*

If the child is eating foods based on the four basic food groups, he is getting all the vitamins he needs. If the child is not eating an adequate diet, vitamin supplements may supply only part of the additional nutrition he needs; protein and needed minerals are not provided by vitamin supplements. Infants usually have vitamin supplements because of their limited diet and until milk consumption can be brought up to one quart of milk a day. Some children may not eat all the foods prepared for them. In such a case, vitamin supplements may help until the child begins to eat an adequate diet. Care must be taken, if supplements are given, not to overdose the child, particularly with Vitamins A and D, which are known to have toxic effects in the body when taken in excessive amounts.

9. *How can a preschooler be encouraged to eat more?*

It is typical for young children to be unpredictable in their eating habits, sometimes eating large amounts of food and other times hardly touching their food. The child's health should be measured by how he looks and feels, not by how much he eats. If the child is getting plenty of rest and exercise and has nourishing, well-prepared meals available to him, he will generally eat what he needs to maintain good health. Also, remember that children eat smaller portions than adults.

10. *What should you do when a child goes on a food jag?*

It isn't unusual for a child to decide he wants to eat only one kind of food for a while. Obviously he will not receive needed nutrition on such jags. But if he has an opportunity to help select foods to eat at mealtime, is not pressured to eat, and has good food available at mealtimes, he will usually get off his jag before his health is impaired.

11. *Is diet more effective than exercise when a person wants to lose weight?*

Authorities agree that the ideal program for weight loss is a combination of regular vigorous exercise and slight food curtailment. If a person engages in such a weight-loss program, 98 percent of the weight loss will be fat. Weight loss by dieting only results in about a 75 percent fat and 25 percent lean body tissue loss. When a person returns to a normal eating pattern, there is a tendency for even greater fat accumulation if lean body tissue has been lost in the dieting process. With the diet/exercise combination, lean body tissue is developed and fat is lost. A person can actually show a loss of inches without showing weight loss because of this development of lean body tissue. Very often the obese person does not eat more than his or her thin counterpart. She or he just moves less.

12. *Can permanent weight loss occur with a special diet, such as a low-carbohydrate high-protein diet or a grapefruit diet?*

The best way for a person to achieve permanent weight loss is to permanently change his or her eating habits. Diets low in carbohydrates, high in protein, and focused on single foods are ultimately dangerous to the body because of the chemical imbalance that usually results. The body is a finely tuned machine acting according to its own complex but unique physical and chemical program. The body needs the proper balance of food elements in order to function at its healthy best. When any of these food elements are missing, the body attempts to make up for the losses by some strange chemical maneuverings. If such diets are prolonged, a person can experience permanent body damage, not permanent weight loss.

13. *Will "spot reducing" occur in areas where I most want to lose weight if I exercise those body areas regularly?*

When you eat a piece of cake or a dish of ice cream or any other calorie-loaded food item, you have no control over where those extra calories are stored in the body. The only thing you control is how many calories you take in and how much energy you expend. If you take in more than you use, you will gain weight. That weight gets stored throughout the body according to your own unique storage formula. However, there are parts of the body that generally store more fat than others, such as the stomach, hips, thighs, and bust in women. If you take in less than the energy you expend, the result will be weight loss. That weight loss occurs in all parts of the body but, fortunate for you, faster in the larger storage areas than in the smaller storage areas. Therefore, a vigorous exercise such as jump rope or running is recommended because it burns up calories faster than a "spot reducing" exercise such as lying on your back and rolling from side to side on your hips. Some muscles of the body, however, may look fat because they are really lacking in strength. Stomach muscles often need strengthening, especially in women, to prevent the "pooched out" look. Exercises suggested in Chapter 2 can help strengthen various body parts. However, if a body area is suffering from too much fat, the general rule is: take in less than you expend in energy and engage consistently in vigorous exercise.

14. *Is it true that a fat baby is a healthy baby and will lose his or her baby fat as he or she grows into childhood?*

Apparently fat cells stored during infancy are affected by either eating patterns established early or by heredity. At any rate, the first year of life seems to be critical in the number of fat cells a person will develop. If a child remains fat at the age of one year, that child will tend to increase the fat cell count in the body until he or she reaches adulthood. In the thin child, the fat cell count changes little between ages two and ten; the fat cells do not change in number when weight gain or loss occurs but are only inflated or deflated. Fifty percent of children with one obese parent grow up to be obese. When both parents are obese, this percentage leaps to 80 percent. It is not clear yet if the eating patterns in the child's environment or the child's heredity determine weight-loss or weight-gain tendencies. A fat baby is not necessarily a healthy baby. Generally, babies eat only until they are satisfied. However, modern high-calorie formulas and high-calorie baby foods mean the modern infant often is taking in many more calories daily than infants did years ago. Most infants until recent times were breast-fed. Breast milk has fewer calories than the same amount of baby formula or baby food. This additional calorie intake may induce the manufacture of more fat cells in the infant of today. These fat cells will always remain in the body, and the older the child grows, the more nutrients these fat cells will require and, thus, the more the person will eat. This contributes to excessive fat. Parents are cautioned to start solids with the infant only when the pediatrician recommends that they do so and to play with babies and keep them active.

15. *Will my stomach shrink after I diet for a few days or weeks?*

The stomach doesn't shrink. However, if you consistently remain on your diet, you will require less food to feel well. In addition, if you stay away from rich foods high in fat and/or sugar content, your body will adjust to not having them. Some people report feeling ill once they start eating rich foods again.

16. *Should family members take supplementary vitamins while on a diet?*

A nutritionally well-balanced diet, which every dieter's should be, does not require food supplements. If a person is on a crash diet, vitamins do not make up for the nutrients not eaten in the food.

17. *If a person consistently stays on a diet, will that person lose weight every week?*

Reaching a plateau is natural when a person is on a diet. This can be due to any number of things including changes in the natural water balance of the body. But eventually a consistent dieter will lose weight again after reaching a plateau.

18. *Does grapefruit burn up fat in the body?*

There is no food that dissolves body fat tissue.

19. *If I eat lots of fish, will this help me lose weight?*

Fish contains less fat and, therefore, has fewer calories than the same amount of meat. However, it is your total daily calorie intake that affects your weight loss, not the type of food you eat.

20. *Is it possible to eat snacks while on a weight-loss diet?*

If snacks are counted as part of the daily weight-loss diet, they can be eaten. Again, what counts is how many calories you eat, not when you eat them. However, it is wise to spread your daily food intake over at least three nutritionally well-balanced meals a day. If you starve yourself all day and then eat all your allotted calories at the evening meal, this may be stoking the engine faster than it can handle the fuel. Thus, the body may store as fat some calories that, had they been eaten at intervals throughout the day, might have been used for body fuel.

21. *Will exercise increase my appetite?*

Vigorous exercise can actually result in lowered appetite because the body is "too tired" to eat. Inactive persons, on the other hand, often seem to have appetites greater than active persons. However, these are the extremes. A person's appetite generally increases or decreases according to the expenditure of energy. This is the body's way of maintaining its weight. Because food is such a strong social reinforcer, the appetite is not the only barometer of the body's need for food. Hunger pangs, extreme fatigue, and nervousness are signals that the body may need food.

22. *Which is easier, to gain weight or to lose it?*

A person trying to gain weight has as much difficulty as a person trying to lose weight. A person who wishes to gain one pound a week must add 500 calories to the daily diet. This can be tough for a thin person.

23. *Is there any reason for an obese person to lose weight if he or she generally feels pretty good?*

Excess weight poses a hazard to adequate functioning of many body systems. Obesity is significantly related to gallbladder diseases, gout, diabetes, hypertension, and cardiovascular disease. It also aggravates chronic conditions such as arthritis and rheumatism. Surgical risk is greater for the overfat person. The mortality rate for obese persons is much higher than for persons of normal weight.

24. *Can I lose weight in a sauna or a steam bath?*

Weight loss a result of a sauna or steam bath is due to water loss through perspiration. Negligible fat is lost. When a person drinks water following a sauna or steam bath, weight loss is replaced.

25. *Does margarine have fewer calories than butter?*

They both have the same number of calories, 100 per tablespoon. Diet margarine has about half the calories of regular butter or margarine.

26. *Should milk be included in a weight-loss diet?*

Milk should be included in the diet unless you are allergic to it. Milk is an excellent source of calcium, protein, and the B vitamins. The recommended milk intake for adults is sixteen ounces per day. With the possible exception of some Vitamin A loss in the butterfat, skim milk has the same nutrients as regular milk but fewer calories.

27. *Can I lose weight by using a vibrating device to break up fat deposits and melt fat away.*

There is no evidence that mechanical devices aid in weight reduction.

28. *Are there some salad oils that have fewer calories than others?*

All salad oils have 125 calories per tablespoon, including safflower, corn, peanut, and olive oil.

29. *Do obese people have gland problems?*

Hardly ever. Blaming glands for an overfat problem is usually a cop-out, a denial of the real problem — eating too much and expending too little.

127

30. *Are people fat because they eat the wrong kinds of food, such as pie or ice cream?*

Not necessarily. Generally the problem is simply eating too much food. If a person consumes more calories than he or she expends, weight gain results.

Part Four

Family Fitness:
Fun and Challenge

An individual's physical capabilities are due, in part, to his or her heritage but to a greater degree to participation and experience after birth. Developing a life-style that encourages participation in physical fitness activities is of vital importance to the health and well-being of each family member, not only during their growing-up years, and lifetimes, but also for the generations yet to come.

Establishing activity areas in the home and surroundings can be beneficial such as: a chin-up bar secured in a doorway or overhead; measuring tape on the wall; scales for weighing; a clock with a second hand for monitoring heart rate; a climbing rope or horizontal ladder placed outdoors or in a recreation room; and other fitness equipment such as trees, fences, etc.

Establishing a tradition of giving birthday and holiday gifts related to fitness is conducive to active participation. Jump ropes, hula hoops, broomsticks, roller skates, ice skates, bicycles, cross-country skis, stationary cycles, family t-shirts and sweat shirts, and other exercise attire is an invitation to a physically active life-style.

The Livewells not only engaged in fitness programs to increase cardiovascular endurance, to limber and strengthen their muscles and joints, and to maintain proper nutrition, but also discovered some games and stunts that could be performed as a family group for fun and friendly challenge. These are activities they can engage in on family nights or on special occasions, such as birthdays and holidays, when friends and relatives come to visit. The Livewells have established a life-style that includes fitness activities as a vital part of their daily lives. Their social activities and even their leisure time at home now includes activities such as those included in this section. Instead of flipping on the television, they engage in activities with jump ropes, broomsticks, bicycles, and roller skates. Individual stunts and partner challenges have become an expected part of family togetherness. These activities focus primarily on flexibility and strength of the muscles, thus helping the family to maintain their fitness programs while at the same time having fun together.

Chapter Seven

Family Challenge
Series

The following activities can bring about increased fitness and provide an element of fun and challenge for family participants.

A. Walk Variations

1. Giant

Purpose: Strength, flexibility of the hip joint.
Description: Progress across the room taking as wide a stride as possible.

2. Tiptoe

Purpose: Strengthen the leg muscles and increase body balance and control.
Description: Rise to a balanced position on the toes and walk around the room maintaining this balance. The ankles are fully extended and the knees remain straight.

3. Ballet Kick

Purpose: Flexibility of the hip joint, strengthen the leg muscles, and increase body balance and control.
Description: Rise to a balanced position on the toes. While maintaining this position, walk around the room, raising the opposite leg as high as possible on each step.

✓4. Toe Grasp

Purpose: Flexibility, balance.
Description: Lean the upper body forward and grasp the toes with the

hands. Walk forward with the weight on the balls and heels of the feet, maintaining the hold on the toes.

5. Toe Touch

Purpose: Flexibility, coordination.
Description: As the right foot steps forward, the left hand reaches forward to touch the right toe. As the left foot steps forward, it is touched by the right hand. Increase the tempo as the individual's ability increases.

6. Heel Touch

Purpose: Flexibility, coordination.
Description: On each step the left hand touches the left heel and the right hand touches the right heel. Increase the tempo as the individual's ability is improved.

7. Crouch Walk

Purpose: Flexibility, leg strength, and balance.
Description: Crouch the body down so the fingers drag on the floor. Maintaining this position, walk forward.

8. Steam Engine

Purpose: Flexibility, coordination.
Description: Clasp the hands behind the head. As the person steps forward on the left foot, the right knee is bent and raised to meet the right elbow; the left elbow and left knee touch on the next step.

9. The Stroll

Purpose: Coordination.
Description: The right foot is brought behind the left leg and progresses forward. The left leg travels behind the right leg and progresses forward.

B. Animal Walks

Individual activities such as animal walks, stunts, and tests of skill are valuable as means of attaining fitness and preparing the body for activities requiring a higher degree of skill.

1. Elephant

Purpose: Flexibility of hamstring muscles.
Description: Bend forward from the hips and waist, keep the knees

straight, clasp the hands together to make the trunk, and reach toward the floor. Move forward keeping the knees straight and swinging the arms back and forth.

2. Bear

Purpose: Flexibility, coordination, strength.
Description: With hands and feet on the floor, progress forward by moving the right hand and right foot and then the left hand and left foot. Perform the skill by progressing forward, moving the right and the left foot at the same time and then the left hand and the right foot at the same time. This is a test of coordination.

3. Monkey

Purpose: Agility, leg strength.
Description: Crouch the body to a monkey position by bending at the hips, knees, and ankles. Keep the weight forward and on the balls of the feet. Move quickly about the area. Scratch the ribs occasionally with the hands.

4. Crab

Purpose: Strength of the shoulder girdle, hands, arms and flexibility of the shoulder joint.
Description: In a position on the hands and feet with the back toward the floor, progress around the room moving in the direction of the head.

5. Lobster

Purpose: Strength of the shoulder girdle, arms and hands, and flexibility of the shoulder joint.
Description: In a position on the hands and feet with the back toward the floor, progress around the room moving in the direction of the feet.

6. Pollywog

Purpose: Strength of the arms, shoulders, back, and ankles.
Description: On the hands and feet in an extended position, move about the room by bending only at the ankle joint. Keep the hips in line with the heels and shoulders.

7. Seal

Purpose: Strength of the shoulder girdle, arms, and hands.
Description: Lie in a prone position with the feet extended. Support the weight on the hands and progress about the room. Keep the head up, let the feet drag on the floor.

8. Inchworm

Purpose: Flexibility of the hamstring muscles, strength of the arms, shoulder girdle, and hands.
Description: In a position on the hands and feet with the hips raised, first move the hands forward as far as the body can extend. Then keeping the legs straight, move the feet forward as flexibility allows without bending the knees. Repeat by moving the hands first and then the feet, measuring as far as possible each time.

9. Chicken

Purpose: Flexibility and coordination.
Description: Stoop forward and grasp the ankles. Maintaining this position, walk around the room.

The following animal walks are very beneficial for developing strength of the leg muscles. It is imperative that they be performed so that the calf of the leg does not press against the back of the upper leg thus putting pressure on the knee cap. This is accomplished by assuming a half-sit rather than a deep-squat position.

10. Duck Walk

Purpose: Leg strength and coordination.
Description: Assume a half-sit position (be sure you do not go below a 90-degree angle). Place the hands on the shoulders and move the arms up and down as you walk around the room.

11. Rabbit Hop

Purpose: Leg strength and coordination.
Description: Assume a half-sit position with the knees and hands on the floor in front of the body. Progress forward by placing the weight on the hands and moving the feet forward. Transferring the weight to the feet, move the hands forward and repeat, progressing around the room.

√ 12. Bunny Hop

Purpose: Leg strength.
Description: Assume a half-sit position, keeping the knees close together and the hands up in the air in front. Push off with the feet to progress forward with little jumps. Do not let the heels touch the buttocks when getting ready to hop.

13. Frog Jump

Purpose: Leg strength and coordination.

Description: Assume a half-sit position with the hands on the floor between the knees. Progress forward around the room by pushing off with both hands and feet to spring in the air.

14. Kangaroo Jump

Purpose: Leg strength.

Description: Assume a half-sit position, keeping the upper body erect and the arms folded in front to assimilate a pouch. Spring as far forward as possible by pushing off with the feet.

C. Combatives

Combative activities test the physical ability of one person against that of another person. Contestants should be equally matched in physical strength, ability, and competitive spirit for maximum benefits to be derived.

The correct body position for all pushing and pulling activities should be:

a. Feet in forward-stride position.

b. Knees bent (for a lower center of gravity).

c. Body leaning in line with the direction of force to be exerted.

Each position allows each person to exert maximum physical strength and eliminate the possibility of strain to the muscles of the back.

1. Hand Pull

Purpose: Strength.

Description: Contestants face each other and grasp hands. Each attempts to pull the opponent over to his own position. Each individual should grasp the wrists of the opponent so that there is a double grasp, with the heel of each person's hands in contact with the other's wrists. This can be varied by having contestants start on one foot, so that they must hop and they pull their opponents.

Variation:

a. Right-hand pull.

b. Left-hand pull.

2. American Wrestle

Purpose: Strength, agility.

Description: Place two contestants so they stand facing each other with chests touching. Each participant places his left arm over the opponent's shoulder, his right arm about the opponent's waist, and touches his own fingers behind the opponent's back. At the signal "go," each contestant attempts to get in back of his opponent with his arms encircling the opponent's waist. After the signal has been given, the original hold may be broken. Either contestant securing the opponent about the waist from behind, whether standing, sitting, lying, or kneeling, wins the bout.

3. Back-to-Back Push

Purpose: Strength.

Description: Place two contestants standing back to back with their elbows locked. Establish a line ten feet in front of each contestant. At the signal "go," each contestant, by pushing backward, attempts to push the opponent over the opponent's baseline. The contestants are not allowed to lift and carry their opponents — pushing only is permitted. Either contestant pushed over his or her own baseline loses the bout.

4. Chinese Jostle

Purpose: Strength, agility, balance.

Description: Place two contestants so they stand facing each other at a distance of five feet. Have each contestant stand on the right foot and clasp the ankle of the left foot with both hands in front of the right thigh. At a given signal, the contestant hops forward and by pushing, lifting, and pressing the uplifted leg and using side-stepping maneuvers against the opponent's uplifted leg, attempts to upset him/her. The contestants do not contact bodies. Either contestant releasing one or both hands or falling to the ground loses the bout. Three out of five bouts determines the winner.

5. Cock of the Walk

Purpose: Strength, agility, balance.

Description: Place two contestants so they stand facing each other at a distance of five feet. The contestants stand on their own right foot holding the left foot behind the body with the right hand. At a given signal, the contestants hop forward. By pushing with the free hand, bucking, side-stepping, and so on, they attempt to overthrow the opponent. The contestants are not allowed to grasp the opponent with the free hand. The contestant placing his or her free foot on the ground or falling to the ground loses the bout. Three out of five bouts determines the winner.

6. Rooster Fight

Purpose: Leg strength, agility, balance.

Description: Two contestants stand within a five-foot circle on the right foot
— the left foot held behind the back with the right hand, the left arm
folded across the body with the left hand on the right shoulder. On a
given signal, the contestants try to force each other out of the circle or
off balance by butting the opponent with the left shoulder. Three wins
out of five determines the winner of the bout.

7. Lifting Contest

Purpose: Strength.
Description: Place two contestants so they stand facing each other with
chests touching. Have each contestant place his/her left arm over the
opponent's right arm and his/her right arm about the opponent's
waist, clasping the hands behind the opponent's back. At the signal
"go," each contestant attempts to lift the opponent from the ground.
The original hold may be broken after the signal to start has been
given. The contestant lifted clear from the ground loses the bout.

ACTIVITIES WITH BROOMSTICKS

The broomstick, sometimes referred to as a wand, is a 30" to 36" piece
of ¾" to 1½" dowling. This has been a popular piece of equipment among
people of all ages as an aid to obtaining physical fitness or gaining physical
prowess.

A. Flexibility

1. Cane Twirling

Purpose: Increase flexibility of the wrist joint.
Description: Grasp the stick in the right hand and rotate it as far around as
possible in either direction. Repeat with the left hand.

2. Over the Head

Purpose: Increase flexibility of the shoulder joint.
Description: Grasp the stick with both hands in an overhand grip. Take the
stick from in front of the body over the head and return without
bending the elbows. Attempt to bring the hands closer together on the
stick with each performance.

3. Shoulder Twist

Purpose: Increase flexibility of the shoulder joint and waist.
Description: Place the broomstick across the upper shoulders with the
crook of the elbow around the ends of the stick. Turn the upper torso of
the body so that the stick is pointing north and south, turn back so that
it points east and west. Repeat to the opposite side. Do 5 to 10 times.

4. Side Bender 1

Purpose: Increase flexibility of the shoulder joint and the waist.

Description: Place the broomstick in the same position as described in number three. Bend to the right side as far as possible keeping the body and the stick in a straight line. Repeat to the left. Do 5 to 10 times.

5. Side Bender

Purpose: Increase flexibility and "tone up" of the waist.

Description: Hold the stick in both hands high above the head. Bend to the right pulling the left arm close to the head and the right arm as far down the right leg as possible. Repeat to the left side with the right arm close to the head and the left arm reaching down the left leg. Repeat 5 to 10 times.

6. Cross Over

Purpose: Increase flexibility of the hip joint and back.

Description: Stand facing the stick. Hold onto the stick with both hands and put it on the floor. Still holding with both hands, step over the stick with both feet and then step back to the original position. You may bend the body at any joint to perform the task, but the hands must hold onto the stick and the stick must remain on the floor.

7. Torso Stretch

Purpose: Increase flexibility of the hip joint and the waist.

Description: Sit in a wide-stride position with the broomstick held in both hands high over the head. Hands approximately thirty to thirty-six inches apart. Twist the upper body so that the right hand extends to touch the left toes. The upper body turns so that you are looking through the window formed by the broomstick and both arms. Return to an upright position and repeat, twisting to the right with the left hand touching the right toes. Repeat 5 to 10 times to each side.

8. Toe Touch

Purpose: Stretch the hamstring muscles.

Description: From a straight standing position with the broomstick held in both hands, reach the stick toward the floor by leaning forward, keeping the knees straight. Move with a smooth continuous movement until stretch pain is felt. Do not let the knees hyperextend. Repeat 5 to 10 times.

9. Through the Stick

Purpose: Total body flexibility.

Description: Hold the stick in front of the body with an overhand grip at each end of the stick.

a. Step the right leg around the outside of the right arm and across the top of the stick.

b. Take the left end of the stick over the head — over the back and to a position where you are straddling the stick.

c. Step over the stick with the left foot. Your arms will be rotated to an inside-out position, but don't let go of the stick with either hand. Complete the task by stepping over the stick with the left foot, take the left end of the stick over the buttocks, across the back, and over the head. Step over the stick with the right foot and you are back to the original position.

B. Strength

1. Finger Walk

Purpose: Develop strength in the fingers, hands, and forearm. Good for strengthening the hands for activities requiring a strong grip such as climbing rope, horizontal ladder, and traveling rings.

Description: Hold the broomstick in one hand with the thumb and little finger on one side and the three middle fingers on the other side. Walk the fingers up the stick and then down the stick without letting the stick slide and without assistance from any other part of the body. Repeat with opposite hand.

2. Pull the Stick

Purpose: Strengthen muscles of hands, arms, chest, and shoulders.

Description: Grasp the broomstick with the hands approximately twelve inches apart. Try hard to pull the stick apart for a count of five — repeat 3 or 4 times with the hands in each of the following positions:

a. Hands held chest high

b. Hands held at hip level

c. Hands held above the head.

Note: Perform the same exercise with both an overhand and an underhand grasp.

3. Push the Stick

Purpose: Strengthen the muscles of the hands, arms, chest, and shoulders.

Description: Follow the directions listed for no. 2 but instead of trying to pull the stick apart, try to push it together, much like an accordion. Repeat in the three positions described above and with both the overhand and the underhand grip.

4. Twist the Stick

Purpose: To strengthen the muscles of the hands and arms.

Description: Grasp the stick tightly so it will not turn in the hands; with the right hand try to turn the stick away from the body, and with the left hand try to turn the stick toward the body giving the feeling of twisting the stick in the middle. Repeat the exercise by turning toward the body with the right hand and away from the body with the left hand. Repeat 5 to 10 times.

5. Grip

Purpose: To strengthen the muscles of the hands, arms, and shoulders and in most events each muscle group of the body.

Description: Both persons grasp the stick with an inside-outside overhand grip. Each person tries to hold the stick steady in his own hands, at the same time trying to turn the stick within his partner's grasp. Start the stick at shoulder level. The winner is determined by succeeding two out of three times. Repeat the exercise with an underhand grip.

6. Touch-down

Purpose: To strengthen the muscles of the hands, arms, and shoulders.

Description: Each person identifies one end of the stick as his end. Take an inside-outside grip with the outside hand about eight to ten inches away from the end of the stick identified as yours. At the signal "go" try to force the opponent's end of the stick to the floor, at the same time keeping your end of the stick off the floor. The winner is determined by touching the opponent's end of the stick to the floor two out of three times.

7. Stick Wrestle

(Note: Make sure you have at least a six-foot square of unobstructed space as this next event can be very vigorous.)

Purpose: To strengthen the muscles of the hands, arms, and shoulders.

Description: Both people grasp the stick with an inside-outside grip. The object of this event is to try to pull, push or twist the stick away from your partner. The winner is determined by succeeding to take the stick away from his partner in two out of three attempts.

8. Partner Tug-o-War

Purpose: To strengthen the muscles of the hands, arms, and shoulders as well as major muscle groups of the body.

Description: Establish a goal line; one person stands in a forward-stride position on one side of the line with his opponent on the other side. The stick is held waist high and directly above the goal line. Each person tries to pull his opponent across the line. (Hands are in an inside-outside overhand position.) Keep your knees bent to insure use of large muscles of the legs rather than the small muscles of the back. Also lower the center of gravity in order to maintain body balance.

9. Partner Pull-over

Purpose: To strengthen the muscles of the arms and shoulders.

Description: Sit on the floor with knees bent and feet touching those of opponent. Grasp the stick with an inside-outside grip directly above the feet. Exerting force by pulling with the hands on the stick and pushing your feet against the opponent's feet, try to pull your opponent to an upright position. Pulling the opponent to his feet two out of three attempts determines the winner.

10. Partner Assist

Purpose: To strengthen muscles of the arms and shoulders.

Description: This is a partner event that requires cooperation rather than competition. Sit on the floor with your knees bent and your feet close to the buttocks. Your partner takes the same position with the toes of his feet touching yours. The stick is held with an inside-outside grip directly above the feet. With an equal pull try to rise to a standing position — both persons rising at the same time.

11. Partner Pull-ups

Purpose: To strengthen muscles of the arms and shoulders.

Description: Person No. 1 lies in a supine position on the floor. Person No. 2 stands astride No. 1 with his feet immediately below the shoulders. No. 2 maintains a stable position by bending the knees and keeping the back straight. No. 2 holds the broomstick as No. 1 pulls his body off the floor so that only the heels are touching. Bring the chin up to the stick and lower 5 to 10 times. Partners reverse positions and repeat the exercise. If the partners are of unequal size, use a threesome — one person to hold at each end of the stick as the third person performs the pull-up. Rotate positions.

Note: Exercise 11 can be done at home by placing a broomstick across two chairs or other stable pieces of furniture and performing the exercise as described for No. 1.

12. Ski Jump

Purpose: Strengthen the leg muscles.

Description: Lay the stick on the floor as an obstacle over which to jump. Assume a half-sit position with the shoulders perpendicular to the stick and the feet pointing toward it. Jump to the opposite side of the stick keeping the shoulders in the same position; by rotating the hips you land with feet again pointing toward the stick. Repeat the exercise rapidly — jumping high in the air each time from the half-sit position.

13. Jump the Stick

Purpose: Increase leg strength, flexibility of the hip joint and back, and practice events leading to increased agility and coordination.

Description: Hold the stick in front of the body with an overhand grip. Jump up in the air, bring the legs to a tuck position and move the stick under the feet before landing. Repeat the same task in reverse by jumping back across the stick in the above fashion. Do not let go of the stick with either hand.

Performance Cues:

    a.   Practice jumping into the air while at the same time pushing the stick down at arms' length.

    b.   Perform this task on a mat or soft-landing surface.

    c.   Practice with a rope or towel may be helpful before trying the stick.

    d.   If your feet do not clear the stick, drop the stick so that you can land on your feet thus preventing a possible accident.

C. Self-testing and Family Challenge

1. Circular Jump

Purpose: Give practice in controlling the body as it changes positions to perform the task.

Description: Grasp the stick at one end with the preferred hand. Move the stick in a circular fashion so that both feet must jump over the stick during each circle. Try the above task by reversing the direction of the circle. Jump with both feet at the same time.

Variation: Have person No. 1 move the stick back and forth changing the tempo of the movement as desired. Person No. 2 jumps the stick each time it is moved. Keep the stick low (one end on the floor). Make sure the partners are facing each other so the jumper can watch the stick at all times.

2. Sword Fight

Purpose: To give practice in quick directional changes in movement of the feet and the hands.

Description: Challenge an opponent who has approximately your same size and physical ability. Each person grasps the end of a broomstick and standing approximately eight feet apart, extends the other end toward his opponent until the two ends meet on the floor. This end of the stick must remain on the floor throughout the performance. On the command "go," each person tries to touch the toes of his opponent while at the same time keeping his opponent's stick away from his own toes. The first person to be touched signifies by saying "touch" or "touché," after which the contest is started over again.

3. Over and Under

Purpose: To give practice in controlling the body as you change body positions from one level to another.

Description: Work in a foursome, two persons hold the broomsticks as the other two perform, then the positions are exchanged. The two broomsticks are held approximately three feet apart — one stick, four feet off the floor, the other about one foot off the floor. The two performers take turns jumping over the low stick and moving under the high stick. After each turn the low stick is raised and the high stick is lowered. Continue this procedure until the participants are no longer able to maneuver the sticks.

Note: Maneuver the sticks as rapidly as possible in order to practice a quick change of position.

D. Coordination

1. Wand Toss

Purpose: To practice eye-hand coordination.
Description:
    a.   Keeping the wand in a perpendicular position, toss it from one hand to the other.
    b.   Holding one end of the stick with the right hand, toss the stick in the air and catch the opposite end with the same hand. Repeat several times with each hand.
    c.   Holding one end of the stick with the right hand, toss the stick in the air and catch the opposite end with the left hand. Repeat by

tossing the stick with the left hand and catching the opposite end with the right hand.

2. Partner Toss

Purpose: To practice eye-hand coordination.
Description:

a. Stand three feet away from a partner and toss the stick from your right hand to your partner's right hand. Keep the stick perpendicular to the floor at all times; this is best accomplished if the hand is placed by the center.

b. Repeat the above using the left hands.

c. Repeat the above tossing from your right to your partner's left.

d. Toss from your right hand to your own left hand, across to your partner's right hand, from the partner's right hand to her own left hand and then back to your right hand to begin the routine again. (The stick travels in a square.) Reverse the direction by starting the toss from left to right.

e. Establish a 4/4 rhythm. Each person holds a broomstick in the center, perpendicular to the floor. On count one the sticks are tossed from the right hand to the individual's own left hand. On count two the sticks are tossed across to the partner's right hand. On count three the sticks are tossed from the right hand to their own left hand; on count four the sticks are tossed from the left hand to the partner's right. Vary the activity by 1) increasing the tempo, 2) reversing the direction, or 3) increasing the distance between partners.

3. Broomstick Footwork

Purpose: To practice eye-foot coordination.
Description:

a. Place two broomsticks on the floor about twelve inches apart. Perform straddle hops by bouncing twice with both feet between the two sticks and once with the feet apart straddling the two sticks. As the feet straddle the sticks the hands clap together over the head. As the feet bounce inside the sticks, the hands are brought down against the thighs.

b. Run through: Place two sticks twelve inches apart and stand with your right side toward the outermost stick. Start the run through with the right foot, bringing the knees up high on each step. On count one place the right foot between the sticks, count two place the left foot between the sticks, count three step outside the stick to the right. Repeat the step pattern placing the left foot inside the sticks on count one, right foot inside on count two, and left foot outside on count three.

c. Hop turn: Step inside the sticks with your right foot; do a hop turn on the right foot and step out left on the left foot. You are now on the opposite side of the sticks from the starting position with the weight on the left foot. Repeat by placing the right foot between the sticks on count one, on count two do a hop turn on the right foot, and on count three step out with the left foot.

Note: Count one and two are performed on the right foot and count three is performed on the left foot. The right foot always performs between the two sticks and the left foot always performs outside the sticks, first to the right and then to the left.

d. The skills described in a, b, and c can become more difficult by performing the skill while the sticks are being moved in a rhythmic pattern. Two persons are designated as beaters — one at each end of the sticks. The beaters are seated so that the feet are doubled back under the buttocks and out of the way of the sticks. The sticks are held, one in each hand, so that the thumb is on one side and the fingers on the opposite side while one surface is in contact with the floor. On counts one and two the sticks are beat against the floor (approximately twelve inches apart). On count three the sticks are brought together in the center. Rotate the hands outward so the surfaces of the sticks can contact each other, thus making a hollow sound as they are struck.

ROPE JUMPING

Rope jumping is one of the most enjoyable and beneficial types of conditioning programs for family members. A jump rope is inexpensive, can be easily stored, taken along on trips, and requires very little space for use. Jump ropes can be purchased that have ball bearings in the handles and allow for smooth and easy turning; however, appropriate lengths of sash cord are suitable and less expensive. The length for each individual can be determined by standing on the rope and bringing the ends to the armpits on each side.

The rope can be used for flexibility and muscle toning as well as for cardiovascular endurance.

A. Flexibility and Muscle Toning

1. Shoulder Rotation

Starting position: Stand erect with rope held taut between hands with arms stretched wide.

Action: Keep the arms straight and the rope taut bring the rope over the head and touch behind. Return to starting postion keeping the arms straight and the rope taut.

Note: As you increase in shoulder flexibility, you are able to bring the hands closer together on the rope.

2. Side Bender

Starting position: Stand erect with feet shoulder width apart and hold the rope taut with arms outstretched above head.

Action: Bend the body to the left side pulling the left arm down to touch the left leg, gently bob for an eight-count set. Perform on each side 1-3 sets.

3. Alternate Toe Touch 1

Starting position: Stand erect with feet in a wide stride, arms above head with rope stretched taut.

Action: Bend the body forward at the hips touching right hand to left foot and stretching left hand high in the air keeping the rope taut. Return to starting position and repeat by touching left hand to right foot. Repeat 10-20 times.

4. Alternate Toe Touch 2

Starting position: Sit erect with legs extended in a wide stride, arms above head with the rope stretched taut.

Action: Reach right hand toward the left foot at the same time rotate the upper torso and hold the rope taut with the left hand high. Return to starting position and repeat by touching the left hand to the right foot. Repeat 10-20 times.

5. Hamstring Stretch 1

Starting position: Stand erect with feet together and knees straight. Fold the jump rope until it is about twelve inches long. Hold taut in hands.

Action: Reach toward the floor for a slow four-second count. Return to starting position and repeat 6-8 times trying to reach further each time.

6. Hamstring Stretch 2

Starting position: Same as hamstring stretch 1.

Action: Reach the hands to the floor and hold the rope taut on the floor. While rocking back and forth from heels to toes, move the rope under the feet and hold behind the heels — move the rope back to the front in the same manner and return to starting position. Repeat 6-8 times, trying to reach behind heels farther each time.

Refer to the jumping-rope activities for cardiovascular endurance described in Chapter 4. These rope-jumping skills not only contribute to cardiovascular endurance, but also to total body toning and leg strength.

Each skill can be used for individual goal setting and for family and neighborhood challenge fun.

ACTIVITIES WITH HOOPS

Hula hoop activities are a challenging way of achieving a state of physical well-being.

1. With hoop tight against back, start hoop circling with a fast forward thrust of the right hand. Rotate body in circular motion against the hoop. Do not twist body. Hoop can be kept in perpetual motion by sideways motion of body, forward and backward motion of body, or circular motion of body.

2. Start at waist (or start at neck), keep hoop circling and work down to knees. To keep circling at knees, hold knees together firmly and point toes in, heels apart, rotating knees in circular motion.

3. Exercises to reduce and improve muscle tone. (a) Bend forward at waist, hang hoop over back of neck. With hands on either side of hoop, roll hoop from side to side on floor. (b) Raise hoop high over head, move body from side to side from the waist up. (c) Hold hoop against back, legs spread apart. Rotate hoop as far as possible in each direction. (Same action starting for twirling around waist.)

4. Family challenge to keep the hoop twirling; keep two or more going at once.

5. Walking Races — see who can walk the fastest, keeping hoop rotating around the waist.

6. Play "Jump the Hoop" — just like jumping a rope.